Journey to Independence

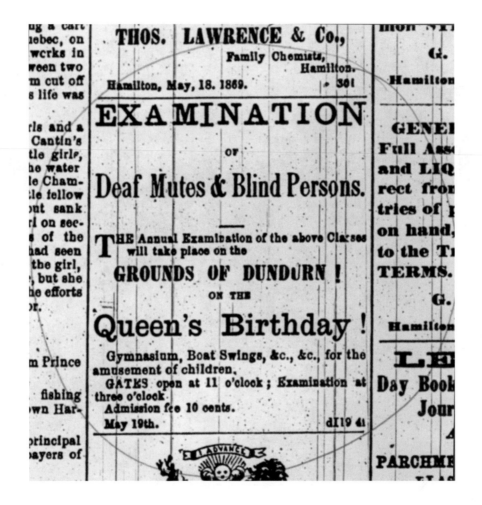

THOS. LAWRENCE & Co.,

Family Chemists,

Hamilton.

Hamilton, May, 18. 1869. 30t

EXAMINATION

OF

Deaf Mutes & Blind Persons.

THE Annual Examination of the above Classes will take place on the

GROUNDS OF DUNDURN !

ON THE

Queen's Birthday !

Gymnasium, Boat Swings, &c., &c., for the amusement of children.

GATES open at 11 o'clock ; Examination at three o'clock

Admission fee 10 cents.

May 19th. dI19 4t

THE CANADIAN NATIONAL INSTITUTE FOR THE BLIND

JOURNEY TO INDEPENDENCE

Blindness ~ The Canadian Story

EUCLID HERIE

THE DUNDURN GROUP
TORONTO

Editor: Elizabeth Duncan
Copy-Editor: Andrea Pruss
Design: Jennifer Scott
Printer: University of Toronto Press

National Library of Canada Cataloguing in Publication Data

Herie, Euclid J.
    Journey to independence : blindness, the Canadian story / Euclid Herie.

Includes bibliographical references and index.
ISBN-10: 1-55002-599-6
ISBN-13: 978-1-55002-599-6

    1. Canadian National Institute for the Blind--History. I. Title.

HV1804.H47 2005   362.4'1'06071   C2005-900174-7

1   2   3   4   5   09   08   07   06   05

Care has been taken to trace the ownership of copyright material used in this book. The author and the publisher welcome any information enabling them to rectify any references or credits in subsequent editions.
        J. Kirk Howard, *President*

Printed and bound in Canada.✪
Printed on recycled paper.
www.dundurn.com

Dundurn Press
8 Market Street, Suite 200
Toronto, Ontario, Canada
M5E 1M6

Gazelle Book Services Limited
White Cross Mills
Hightown, Lancaster, England
LA1 4X5

Dundurn Press
2250 Military Road
Tonawanda, NY
U.S.A. 14150

CNIB gratefully acknowledges the sponsorship of Canadian Ophthalmological Society, Canadian Association of Optometrists and Novartis Ophthalmics

  We acknowledge the support of the **Canada Council for the Arts** and the **Ontario Arts Council** for our publishing program. We also acknowledge the financial support of the **Government of Canada** through the **Book Publishing Industry Development Program** and **The Association for the Export of Canadian Books**, and the **Government of Ontario** through the **Ontario Book Publishers Tax Credit** program, and the **Ontario Media Development Corporation**.

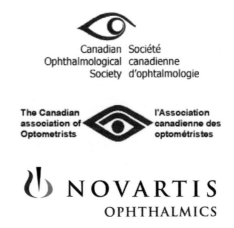

Canadian Ophthalmological Society / Société canadienne d'ophtalmologie

The Canadian association of Optometrists / l'Association canadienne des optométristes

NOVARTIS OPHTHALMICS

... The Past

To my mother, Annette Marie Guenette
(April 20, 1912–August 5, 1962),
St. Jean-Baptiste, Manitoba.

For love and inspiration rising above poverty
and illiteracy to her graduation as a teacher
from the Normal School at Brandon, Manitoba,
in the mid-1930s despite the very depth of the
Great Depression. This work is to honour her
memory with enduring gratitude.

... The Future

To my three granddaughters, Gabriel Sarah
(April 19, 1997), Madeleine Ellen (November 12,
1998), and Charlotte Annette (April 10, 2001).

They are together and as individuals a source
of unending delight and a joy to all our family.
Their noisy youthfulness, wonderful talent, and
humour are a soothing influence and great
reassurance for a future of hope and promise.
May they discover knowledge and some of life's
lessons in this *Journey to Independence*.

TABLE OF CONTENTS

FOREWORD

The book you are about to read will take you on a journey that touches on four centuries. Over the course of it, you will meet some extraordinary, passionate men and women, most of them blind, who worked with tireless determination to make this country a better, more accepting place for Canadians who are blind, visually impaired, or deaf-blind.

You will meet the founders of the Canadian National Institute for the Blind, an organization that was started by a dedicated group of seven men, including two war-blinded soldiers, at the end of the First World War. And although the war was certainly the catalyst in the creation of the CNIB, it most likely would have happened anyway, as the natural evolution of the library for the blind and schools and associations for the blind that existed at that time.

You will also see how Canadian attitudes towards blindness have changed over the years, and you will, realize, I hope, that although we've come a long way, we still have far to go.

You will learn that blind people, like all people with disabilities, do not need sympathy — they need equal access to education, oppor-tunity, employment, and empower-ment. The people you are about to meet will tell you that, in their own words. This is, after all, their story. Our story.

For me, the CNIB isn't just a well-established Canadian institu-tion with historic and philanthrop-ic importance. It has personal relevance. You see, I was blinded in my left eye during Second World War combat, and my remaining vision is now failing, so I am not just a supporter of the CNIB but also one of its 105,000 clients. I am grateful every day for its help on my own journey to independence.

I hope you will enjoy this read-able, remarkable, and unusual approach to Canadian history, which took three years to research and write. I believe it will serve for quite some time as a resource on blindness in this country.

The Honourable Barnett (Barney) Danson, P.C., O.C. Toronto, Ontario November 2004

ACKNOWLEDGEMENTS

Alex Saunders, CNIB consultant on rehabilitation from the late 1940s to his retirement in the 1960s, recorded a number of candid interviews with CNIB executives, usually after their retirement, including Art Weir, Doug Strong, Grace Worts, Art Magill, and Bill Milton because, he said, "Someday, somebody will want to write a book on our history." Well, here it is.

On the sixtieth anniversary of the CNIB in 1978, Paul O'Neill recorded over 130 detailed interviews with staff and volunteers across Canada. Dayton Forman and Joan Keagy ensured that these precious recollections were meticulously preserved and transcribed. Over three years I added another fifty or so personal interviews to the collection. This recorded treasury is both delightful to listen to and informative. Everyone interviewed revealed amazing insight and passion for the CNIB and its mission. At least half of these folks are now deceased, and we owe each of them a vote of thanks and remain in their debt.

Nancy Ind, niece and literary executor of Marjory Wilkins Campbell, E.A. Baker's official biographer, graciously gave permission for the unedited interviews with Baker to be dubbed from reel-to-reel-tapes to cassette for my personal reference. Nancy also shared her aunt's diary and the original manuscript for *No Compromise*. Thanks, Nancy, for your support and encouragement.

In a reference I once described Amie Kiddle as a "star." Amie worked for over a year with me to source volumes of written data upon which we built this manuscript. Thanks, Amie, for slogging through all forty-four boxes in the National Archives and fifty years' worth of CNIB archives and minute books. Not only did she glean much good stuff, but with her high energy and intense focus she was a tremendous help.

Over the winter of 2002 at Chris Blazie's Florida house, Lida Kotzar and I got down to some serious writing, and the first two chapters are much as we drafted them.

I want to recognize the CNIB executive directors who were always willing to assist whenever asked.

Noted broadcaster and author Pete McGarvey, of Leacock and Orillia fame, not only inspired me to do this history but led us to Kirk Howard and the Dundurn Group. Pete, you've always been a great friend.

It was when Gary Homer of Calgary was the national chair that we first seriously discussed — during long flights on World Blind Union business and train rides to Montreal — the importance of writing this history. Gary supported the idea from the outset, went to bat for the financing, and maintained a personal interest in the project. Thank you, Gary.

I also thank his successor, Frances Cutler of Ottawa, for a seamless transition and her unending encouragement. Fran was my most enthusiastic reader with candid suggestions. Her demands to know "What comes next?" sent me back to the talking computer.

St Dunstan's in England, the Sir Arthur Pearson Association, and a dozen organizations in North America, Australia, and New Zealand collaborated with reference material.

Acknowledgements

I sincerely thank the members of the book's advisory group, beginning with its chair, Eugene Lechelt, who could not have been more supportive or generous with his time. Other members of the group include Patricia Dirks, retired professor of history (Brock University, St. Catharines), who rummaged through the Victoria Archives and recruited Shirley Tillotson. A renowned historian and professor at Dalhousie University, Halifax, specializing in Canadian philanthropy, Shirley's input and guidance were always spot on. Shirley has the rare gift of being able to offer gentle criticism with aplomb.

Our committee scribe was Barbara Marjeram, who dedicated whatever time she could steal away from her CNIB duties to organize the CNIB archival holdings in Toronto. Earlier, Grace Worts, assisted by Betty Milton, had classified and arranged for the written records of the institute from its founding in 1918 to 1980 to be transferred to the National Archives in Ottawa. The material that remained in Toronto was in a frightful condition. Under Barbara's leadership, Anik Cardinal, Joanne Mackie, and Katherine Calleja brought considerable order to the written and photographic materials. Thanks to them, sourcing materials was considerably easier than it might have been. Barbara also served as the key liaison person with our publisher, the Dundurn Group, and has earned our thanks.

From the advisory group I come last to Richard Huyda, a lifelong friend, author, and specialist in Canadian history and photography with the National Archives. Richard has been a CNIB volunteer, taking a special interest in our archives, for a number of years. He spent untold time and energy, which included trips from Ottawa, making helpful suggestions to improve the manuscript. I thank him for his encouragement and thank his wife, Elaine, for sharing him with us.

Beloved Canadian author Roch Carrier (*The Hockey Sweater*) offered quiet encouragement and showed me by example the kind of patience an author needs. During his term as Librarian at the National Library, I believe he came to appreciate the issue of accessible information.

When the work was beginning to stall, we recruited Elizabeth Duncan, a former CNIB communications manager, who had drafted speeches for me at the CNIB. Elizabeth came on board at chapter three, and together we wrote, edited, rewrote, and edited yet again. She also spent hours in the CNIB archives sourcing colour material and did the fact checking. I'm grateful to her for agreeing to write chapter thirteen on my years as president and CEO. It is her work alone. As the manuscript grew, we spent long hours on it together during train rides to Montreal, at the Albany and Halifax clubs, and at my kitchen table. We will remain friends and colleagues, of that I'm certain.

Elizabeth particularly wanted to thank her friend and colleague, longtime CNIB employee Carol Putt, for her editorial support and expertise.

Thanks to Craig Lillico and Jennifer Hendren for processing invoices and keeping me on budget. Dick Hale-Sanders came on board immediately after he was elected national chair in 2003. His question, "What's the message?" kept me focused. "The book should entertain, inform and hold the reader's interest," he would remind me. Well, Dick, in the interests of fairness and balance, I was sometimes gentler and more measured in my narrative than I wanted to be. I would be very pleased, however, if the book comes somewhere near what you wanted it to.

Another Dick, Richard Smith of Winnipeg, served as Manitoba's division chair in Manitoba and as national chair from 1980 to 1983. Currently honorary chair of the institute, Dick, who loves to recount how he recruited me in 1977 from the Children's Aid Society of Winnipeg, was with me every step of the way, as was Don Ross.

Barney Danson enthusiastically accepted my invitation to write the foreword to this book. I am honoured to have such a good friend say kind words of encouragement and support. Himself an author, Barney is a most distinguished Canadian who is held in high esteem and affection by all who know him. Barney, on behalf of all of us, thank you for this and for so much more you do every day toward the advancement of blind persons in Canada.

Acknowledgements

For twenty-seven years, Jim Sanders and I worked side by side at both the CNIB and in the World Blind Union. From 1983 until my retirement, Jim reported to me. Now he serves in the top post. Former CNIB presidents Ross Purse and Robert Mercer join me in encouraging and supporting Jim, knowing only too well the hidden demands and confidentialities of the president's office. All the more reason that I owe Jim a special debt of gratitude for his guidance, support and encouragement. On his young watch Jim already has a digital library, a new national service center, and now a history book to his credit.

In the end, current and former members of the national board hold the ultimate responsibility for this work. Although I cannot thank each of them here, I will always be grateful for their endorsement and for voting the financial resources for the project.

There are also many others, too numerous to mention, in every corner of this wonderful land, who held my hand and urged me forward. I thank all of you, and hope you will enjoy this book and share it with others.

With deep personal gratitude.

Euclid Herie, C.M., M.S.W., LL.D.
CNIB President Emeritus

INTRODUCTION

Invitations to examine the progress of blind students by way of a public spectacle were not unusual in the late nineteenth century. In those days, such events were a necessary part of maintaining a designated educational institution and were justified on the grounds of heightening public awareness. People who were blind were sheltered in homes or institutions, and their appearance in public was more of a curiosity than a natural occurrence.

However, it is entirely possible that this examination was cancelled because of a disaster that had occurred the day before:

A new residence for blind students, Earlham Cottage, at Mrs. Terrell's Emerald Street home in Hamilton, Ontario, burned to the ground on May 18, through the ignorance and carelessness of a deaf-mute boy who placed some hot ashes in a pail in the stable. The pupils barely escaped. If it had not been for the noble bravery of Miss M. McGann many might have lost their lives, as it was a most difficult task to get the frightened children out of their beds.

The 1869 fire on Emerald Street occurred in an era of Canadian history that experienced a shift in attitudes and legislation in public policies toward education and welfare. During those years, significant rights and freedoms for blind people were woven into the legislative, judicial, and cultural fabric of Canadian society. The education and training of blind students in twenty-first-century Canada is dramatically different from those early years, which is a proud reflection of this altered socio-political environment.

CANADA — ITS ORIGINAL INHABITANTS

References to blindness can be found in the oral traditions and hieroglyphics of Canada's Aboriginal, Inuit, and Metis peoples. Perhaps these tribal and family traditions were thought to protect and nurture those who were born blind or became blind through disease or accident. Infant mortality and disease, combined with the harsh demands of a nomadic existence, may have exacted other solutions for those unable to survive and contribute without strength and good health, including the use of sight.

Archival and anecdotal references recorded by early settlers, religious orders, and trading companies in the New World may well make reference to blindness, either among their own membership or in the population at large. This narrative does not attempt to address this phase of Canada's evolution. Rather, it concentrates on a historic era where the demographic shift in population and changing values grew out of not only the Industrial Revolution but also a gradual transformation to an urban society.

CONFEDERATION AND BEYOND

The changes that have been made in public policy, legislation, and awareness with respect to blindness and visual impairment have been led not so much by politicians as by public outcry and concerted advocacy on the part of individuals and private organizations. Two world wars in the first half of the twentieth century left a profound legacy that would affect the lives of the war-blinded in every country, setting in motion a genuine renaissance of attitudinal and legislative change and previously unimagined service programs for blind people of all ages — in sharp contrast to the responses to disability and blindness resulting from armed conflict that had formerly appeared throughout civilization. These developments, preceded by the movement for free public education, would eventually include blind people and result in early efforts to develop organized services for blind Canadians. The prolonged and ongoing evolution is truly unique to Canada and relates directly to our growth as a nation.

Canadian Confederation, as defined through the British North America Act and its subsequent amendments, set out a clear delineation of provincial rights and powers and was designed with the expectation that the provinces of Canada would govern and coexist in harmony with one another. At the same time, Confederation recognized the central role and powers of the federal government. Those early decisions and the delicate jurisdictional balance of powers between the Parliament of Canada and the provincial and territorial governments became a blueprint that shaped and continues to have a profound influence on services for blind and visually impaired Canadians.

It has been a long journey from the period in Canadian history when blind people were relegated to poverty, derision, pity, abuse, and social conditions that, with few exceptions, left them with a bleak promise for the future. What made the journey possible for many blind Canadians was the development of a national service organization for the blind, the Canadian National Institute for the Blind (CNIB). On March 30, 1918, the CNIB received a federal charter as a charitable organization from the government of Canada. From this modest beginning, the contributions of strong leaders and a committed corps of volunteers empowered the CNIB to achieve successes far beyond the vision of its seven founders and their associates. Viewed on a national scale, the range of services at the heart of today's Canadian National Institute for the Blind is truly unique and, some might suggest, a remarkable working model of the Canadian confederacy.

The men who crafted the CNIB's charter and constitution provided a sphere of influence and leadership that would stretch beyond Canada's borders. This book will guide its readers to an understanding of the development of this unparalleled national organization. What follows is an account of an amazing experiment in Canadian philanthropy — a story that must be told.

CHAPTER 1
Education and Training

THE INVENTION OF BRAILLE AND EARLY EDUCATION

The seeds for organized services for the blind were planted during Canadian Confederation, and the Canadian National Institute for the Blind that exists today has grown from roots buried deep within the traditions and challenges of our young nation. Then, as now, Canada consisted of a diverse population spread over an enormous geographic landscape. Linguistic and cultural traditions somewhat shaped by religious influences were inexorably woven into the early educational and service programs for blind youth. Canada's proximity to the United States and historic ties to France and Great Britain created an ideal environment to support, shape, and influence policies and legislation on the quality of life for citizens who were either blind or threatened with blindness.

In the years leading up to 1867 and Confederation, education, welfare, and cultural responsibilities were recognized as falling within the purview and jurisdiction of the then four provinces. It is therefore not surprising that three institutions for the education of the juvenile blind were established in three of those provinces: Ontario, Quebec, and Nova Scotia. No reference has been found in the early literature to suggest that blind and visually impaired Canadians would one day be served by a national organization.

Schools for the blind in Canada followed a natural evolution from what had already been developed in early nineteenth century Europe and other parts of the world. In 1785, Valentin Haüy, a French philanthropist, introduced formal education for the blind in Paris when he provided instruction to the first pupil, François Lesueur. Within a decade, Britain, Germany, Austria, and Russia followed, organizing educational institutions specifically designed for instructing people without sight. By the mid-nineteenth century other countries had adopted a similar pattern, including the United States of America; in Boston, Massachusetts, the New England Asylum for the Blind (later renamed the Perkins School for the Blind) received its charter in 1829.

From the beginning, teaching and training blind pupils focused on reading and writing as well as on providing instruction in music and various manual arts and trades. The biggest challenge was determining how to teach students who couldn't see well enough to read print. Instruction using embossed books of Roman script in Europe (Gothic script in the United States) was the first method to be adopted. It was believed that this method would parallel the teaching of reading and writing skills to people with sight and would enable sighted instructors to instruct using a familiar medium.

By 1830, Louis Braille's six-dot alphabet had begun to gain wide acceptance. Relatively simple to learn but complex in its numerous applications, braille opened a new world for blind students. Nevertheless, despite braille's many obvious advantages, there was resistance, and it was many years before it achieved recognition as a medium equal to print. Readers interested in the history of braille might wish to read *Braille into the Next Millennium*.

Moon type, a form of embossed raised script developed and named after its nineteenth-century English inventor, Dr. William Moon, was considered easier to read with the fingers than either braille or raised print. Later, the United States developed the New York Point method of raised dots to add to this tactile Tower of Babel. Whether desirable or not, the proliferation of tactile systems provided the means for education, allowing blind people everywhere to communicate with one another and with the sighted public. From ancient times until the invention of braille, blind people had been, with the exception of oral teachings, confined to a world of ignorance and illiteracy. Braille, as a new literacy tool, provided blind people with access to education and the chance to pursue newfound freedoms and independence.

Canada's institutions and emerging forms of government in the first half of the nineteenth century were slow to recognize the educational and social needs of blind people. In 1852 in Canada West (renamed Ontario in 1867), the first evidence is found of the government's intent to introduce legislation and allocate resources in an early effort to recognize and remedy social injustices and pro-

vide educational programs for blind citizens. These first initiatives were likely based on prior experience from similar programs in the United States and Europe. By the early 1860s, special schools for the blind in Canada were modelled on foreign programs.

In most countries throughout the world, including Canada, modern schools for the blind bear little resemblance to the early models. The early Canadian solution for dealing with people who were blind or deaf was to define them legisla-

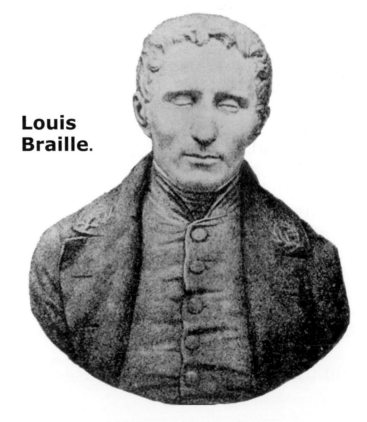

Louis Braille.

tively as individuals deserving to be housed and protected by legislative provisions dealing with prisons and asylums. The blind person, although perhaps not identified as criminal or insane, was nevertheless categorized as a public charge and deemed worthy of charitable or institutional care that in many respects was also custodial.

In an address to the Convention of the American Association of Instructors for the Blind in July of 1932, Dr. J.A. Macdonald offered the following perspective on the nineteenth-century view of a blind Canadian:

> … you must realize what the conditions of the English speaking Canadian blind were prior to 1873. Few, if any, sightless persons were then earning their own living; the great majority were either housed within the four walls of inhospitable asylums, or eked out a miserable existence by begging. They were in very truth "prisoners in dark towers" awaiting a Childe Roland to free them from captivity.

In Quebec, the same attitudes and conditions prevailed for the adult blind, while many blind children were placed in orphanages.

EDUCATION IN ATLANTIC CANADA

These attitudes are also consistent with the decision made by the government of Nova Scotia in 1867 to build the Halifax Asylum for the Blind at a cost of $14,000. This decision was due, in large part, to the initiative and generosity of a Nova Scotia businessman, Scottish-born William Murdoch, who bequeathed £5,000 toward the funding of an institute for the blind. For four years, the institution functioned more as an asylum than a school. However, the charisma and persistence of a blind educator, Charles Frederick Fraser, born in Windsor County, Nova Scotia, and educated at the Perkins School for the Blind in Boston, gradually changed the institution's role and definition to emphasize education and training as opposed to custodial tradition. Finally, in 1882, after repeated requests, the Nova Scotia legislature dropped the reference to an asylum and amended the legislation to adopt a change of name to the School for the Blind. This renaming action represented a major shift in public policy and a growing awareness of the value and meaning of education and training for blind students.

This change was neither an accident of history nor spontaneous enlightenment on the part of the government. Frederick Fraser, appointed principal of the school in 1873, wanted to help the blind "... to be free by training them to earn their own livelihood."

An excerpt from Mary McNeil's article, "The Blind Knight of Nova Scotia: Sir Frederick Fraser," gives us a glimpse of Sir Frederick Fraser's tenacity and determination. In 1881, to establish free education for the blind, he launched a concerted campaign to visit each of Nova Scotia's fourteen counties:

Nothing daunted, he procured a horse and wagon and started out on his long tour of eleven hundred miles. He took with him several teachers and the orchestra of the school and gave concerts. For forty-five consecutive nights he addressed audiences on the claim of the blind. On his return to Halifax, he went again to the Legislature, armed with all the resolutions. The glorious result of the campaign was an Act of Parliament Giving Free Education for the Blind of Nova Scotia — in 1882! In this he led America.

In part, the Act read:

(1)   The parent or guardian of any blind person between the ages of six and twenty-one years, who has, under the provision of "The Poor Relief Act," a settlement in any municipality, city or town, may apply to the warden of such munici-

pality or to the mayor of such city or town, for an order for the admission of such person into the Halifax School for the Blind, which order the said warden or mayor shall at once grant under his hand and the corporate seal of the municipality city or town, on being satisfied that such blind person is between the ages above prescribed, and has a legal settlement in such municipality, city or town.

(2)   Pupils entering the school between the ages of six and ten years shall be entitled to remain several years in addition to the time in attendance under ten years of age; those entering between the ages of ten and thirteen years shall be entitled to remain seven years;

those entering between the ages of thirteen and seventeen years shall be entitled to remain five years; those entering between the ages of seventeen and twenty-one years shall be entitled to remain three years.

(3)   For every blind person received into the Halifax School for the Blind under an order from the warden of any municipality or under an order from the mayor of a city or town which contributes to the Municipal School Fund, and educated and boarded therein, the Board of Managers of such school shall be entitled to receive from the Provincial Treasury the sum of six hundred dollars per annum, payable half-yearly, and also

to receive annually the sum of six hundred dollars, payable yearly, from the Municipal School Fund of such municipality.

Other provincial governments had made earlier moves to enshrine the right to a free public education for all sighted children, but enormous credit is due to the Nova Scotia legislators who alone had the courage and foresight to legislate this right for blind youth. In this respect they led the way in Canada, removing the ambiguity of general rights and freedoms and placing the blind residents of Nova Scotia on an equal basis with all of its citizens. The government of New Brunswick adopted similar legislation in 1892.

Sadly, in several provinces, generations of blind youth would have to wait for decades to be assured of the same right.

But the living conditions were often difficult for the children. In the 2003 documentary *City in Ruins*, the narrator introduces journalist and author Robert MacNeil, who is best known as the co-host of the *MacNeil/Lehrer NewsHour* on PBS.

As a choir boy in 1940s Halifax, Robert MacNeil watches as the residents of a school for the blind make their uncertain way to their places in the front pews.

"I remember they were so shabbily dressed," MacNeil says, "and their hair was so messily cut on the assumption, I suppose, that they wouldn't notice because they were blind. They would hold onto each other to know when to rise and when to kneel and look up with strange-angled faces towards the light coming from the stained glass windows."

Robert Mercer, managing director of the CNIB from 1980 to 1983, was sent to the Halifax School in the 1950s at the age of eight and remained there until he graduated, having completed Grade 11. He remembers that classes were small, weekends were loosely structured, and that although his home was just four hundred kilometres away, in Sydney, he was allowed home only at Christmas and for the summer holidays.

"I was told later that I was one of the most difficult cases of homesickness," he recalled in a 2004 interview. "I had been separated from my parents and nine brothers and sisters, so it was really tough. Sending me there was a difficult choice for my parents. It was either send Robert away to school, or he doesn't get an education."

In her book *Reading Hands: The Halifax School for the Blind*, Shirley Trites provides a detailed account of the school's history. Located on Murdock Square, facing University Avenue, the school was renamed Sir Frederick Fraser School in 1977 and was demolished in 1983.

EDUCATION IN QUEBEC

Education of the blind in the province of Quebec predates the decisions made by the government of Nova Scotia and pursued an entirely different course. In this province, the Roman Catholic Church and its religious orders played a leading role in the development of social and educational programs for the poor and indigent residents of the province.

In Quebec and elsewhere in the young Canadian nation, the majority of blind children and adults were cared for, and likely protected by, immediate and extended family members.

Other blind people — those not left to beg on the street or live in orphanages and asylums — were accommodated by various means, mostly by female religious orders. The exception to this was the establishment of an elementary school by the Montreal Association for the Blind following its founding in 1909.

In 1861, a visually impaired priest, Father Benjamin Victor Rousselot, approached the Sisters of Charity (the Grey Nuns) with the request that they consider accepting blind pupils for training and education. The provincial government seemed content to leave the question of education of blind youth to the nuns, and the

Nazareth Asylum was established in Montreal. Within a year, the asylum admitted its first pupils and was renamed L'Institut Nazareth. Susanne Commend's history of the institution, *Les Instituts Nazareth et Louis-Braille, 1861–2001: Une Histoire de Coeur et de Vision*, published in 2001, spans the 140 years from the founding of L'Institut Nazareth and provides an incisive and detailed account of the development of services and education in Quebec.

The provincial government provided only sporadic grants to L'Institut Nazareth, and the nuns struggled constantly to find financial support from within their order, from families of the students, and from the general public. Despite this struggle, there is little doubt that those students fortunate enough to be admitted to the school received a high calibre of education with a strong emphasis on music and the theatre. Less gifted students had the option of learning trades and were gradually phased into mainstream Quebec society.

A major advantage to establishing a progressive educational and industrial training program in Montreal was the direct linguistic interchange with the well-established blind organizations in Paris, France. This permitted the recruitment of highly qualified music teachers from France and allowed students to benefit from knowledge and experience that dated to the beginning of the nineteenth century.

In 1865, L'Institut Nazareth received its first braille book from the National French School in Paris. From the outset, the Grey Nuns opted for the braille alphabet and music notation developed by Louis Braille; soon, books in French braille began to circulate in Quebec. This decision avoided the confusion that ensued among English-speaking schools for the blind that adopted varying, and at times competing, embossed systems. For example, the Halifax School adopted raised letters in 1875 but introduced Moon type only two years later, establishing a circulating library for its students and the adult blind in 1879. Brantford's Ontario Institution for the Blind adopted the American New York Point system in around 1900. With this diverse approach, it is small wonder that literacy of the blind of Canada and access to materials for gaining knowledge remained issues for more than a century and a half.

It is worth noting that in Quebec, the Catholic and Protestant faiths were largely divided along linguistic lines between French and English. L'Institut Nazareth admitted both males and females who, with very few exceptions, were French-speaking Roman Catholics, and it operated very much like a convent in that the students were expected to practise their faith and participate in the daily maintenance of the school. As it was a residential facility, the boys and girls were segregated as much as possible and housed separately.

For nearly eighty years the school flourished and attendance grew. The curriculum was under the direct supervision of the Montreal Catholic School Board and paralleled the quality of education among the general population. The first major difficulty for the school arose from a little-known but significant provision that prohibited female religious orders from caring for and educating boys over the age of twelve. As the pattern of

admissions changed, and the demands for higher education grew, the Grey Nuns became increasingly reluctant to care for and educate over-age male students. They repeatedly sought to persuade the leadership of the Roman Catholic Church, including the Cardinal of Montreal, to take action and establish a school for adolescent boys. They also appealed fervently to male religious orders to take on this responsibility, even going so far, in 1912, as to offer them an inducement of $75,000 for this purpose. For an entire generation, blind boys over the age of twelve, with few exceptions, were denied an education because of this regulation.

Most blind males above the age of twelve were forced to remain at home, although the Montreal Association for the Blind accepted a few of these boys, as did the MacKay Institute for Deaf Mutes, founded in about 1870 by Joseph MacKay, a member of one of Montreal's most prominent Scottish families.

For the most part, though, only those few boys whose families were resourceful or wealthy could continue their education at schools for the blind in Halifax, Brantford, or the United States.

In 1953, the situation took a turn for the better when an order of Roman Catholic brothers, aided by a grant from the provincial government and resources from the Grey Nuns, opened the L'Institut Louis Braille on Claremont Street in Montreal for boys above the age of twelve.

Unfortunately, the school could accommodate only fifty boarders, when there were more than one hundred potential students. This injustice was not finally resolved until 1960, when L'Institut Louis Braille moved to modern, spacious premises on Beauregard Street on Montreal's south shore.

Meanwhile, in 1940, L'Institut Nazareth had moved to larger quarters on Queen Mary Road, but the outbreak of the Second World War coincided with the next major obstacle L'Institut Nazareth would have to overcome. The school was essentially bankrupt, so it leased the Queen Mary Road facility to the federal government, which used it as a flight training school, and the Grey Nuns relocated, with their students, to smaller premises. L'Institut Nazareth continued

to educate boys under twelve until the Grey Nuns finally closed their school in June 1975. In September 1975, the two schools, L'Institut Nazareth and L'Institut Louis Braille, merged, and Les Instituts Nazareth et Louis Braille (INLB) was established as the primary school for the blind in the province of Quebec, with direct links to the provincial government and a more secure funding base. The school's existence was short-lived, however, and the institution became a rehabilitation centre in 1976 with the subsequent addition of braille and audio library programs. In Quebec, as in other provinces, the mainstreaming of blind children into public schools was becoming a reality.

Although this is not a criticism of the education of the blind in Quebec, the establishment of the three other major schools for the blind in Canada under the auspices of the provincial governments resulted in far more equitable treatment of the blind than in Quebec, ensuring that all blind pupils were guaranteed a basic education.

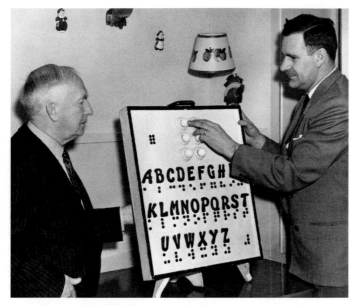

In an undated photo, Fern Huneault of the Quebec division of the CNIB demonstrates a braille teaching aid.

EDUCATION IN ONTARIO

The intervention of provincial politicians in the education of the blind in Ontario was recorded as early as 1845. This coincides with the growing acceptance that public education should be available to all children as a basic right and should be funded from the public purse.

In fairness, the provincial legislators of Canada West, although slow to move, were not entirely without conscience or vision. After the government sent Rev. Dr. Egerton Ryerson, chief superintendent of education for Canada West, on a visit to schools in Europe to inspect their education systems, Ryerson engineered the Common School Act of 1846, which provided free education for all children, and adopted his great principle that "every child in the land has the right to such an education as will make him a useful member of society." The act paved the way for the education of the blind, but, as noted earlier, this would take another twenty-five years.

In 1852, the Legislative Assembly of Canada West voted $80,000 toward the construction of an asylum for blind and deaf people. In 1854, another allocation of $20,000 was voted, but in neither instance was a facility ever constructed. Archival material and recorded proceedings from this period in Canadian legislative history are difficult to source, in part because Parliament was located in several cities over the years and in part because some documents were destroyed by fire. It is clear, however, from research that the legislators definitely intended to build facilities, using public funds, for the education and training of the blind, but it was not until 1869 that these good intentions were actually acted upon. In the meantime, through the initiative of private individuals, Canada West's first and only private school for the blind was established.

In 1857, F.J. Campbell, a teacher at the Institute for the Blind in Wisconsin, wrote a letter to the mayor of Toronto, John Beverley Robinson, proposing to open an institute for educating the blind in Canada.

> Canada — having a population of nearly two million, must, according to the most reliable statistics, have from one thousand five hundred to two thousand blind, several hundred of whom must be suitable subjects for school.
>
> Shall this unfortunate class grope their way any longer in mental as well as physical darkness or shall the veil which obscures their moral and mental vision be withdrawn? ... I propose to open an institution for the Education of the Blind in Canada. I address you on the subject because I believe Toronto to be the best point to locate ... It will be necessary ... for your citizens to make the first move; and then call upon the general government for its assistance.

This early offer of cooperation by an American was an indicator of heightened awareness and may well have served as an impetus to establishing the private school that finally opened in Toronto the following year.

It was Irish immigrant John Barrett McGann, though, who undoubtedly created the greatest push toward the development of this new school. Arriving in Toronto in the summer of 1855, McGann was an educator, author, philanthropist, and fierce advocate for people who were called in those days "deaf-mutes." As a result of his persistent labours, a school for deaf and blind students was opened at the Phoebe Street Schoolhouse in Toronto in June 1858. Indeed, the Phoebe Street Schoolhouse might well be considered the first educational institution for the blind in Canada. Funding for the school appears to have come from a combination of ongoing private contributions and a gradual infusion of public grants.

The practice of combining deaf and blind people in an educational institution was not a new one, either in North America or elsewhere, and was repeated in other provinces in Canada. In Quebec, for example, the two groups were brought together for care and education at the Mackay Institute, but only for a short period, while in British Columbia, the government insisted on a combined educational program for students who were blind or deaf.

For eleven years, McGann operated his school with fewer blind students than deaf. In 1862, it was reported that there were four blind students compared to twenty who were deaf. By 1864, the sixth annual report of the Upper Canada Institution for the Deaf and Dumb and for the Blind stated, "... during the past year there were fifty-three pupils in attendance, forty-seven of whom are deaf mutes and six blind."

McGann deserves enormous credit for his unrelenting efforts and fierce advocacy. Although chiefly focused on deaf people, he recognized the needs and entitlements of blind students and young adults. In the late 1860s, he petitioned the government of Ontario on behalf of six hundred parents who described their blind children as "our most unfortunate charges."

In 1864, McGann experienced political intrusion first-hand. That year, a Dr. Ryan of Hamilton, Ontario, in the guise of the school's medical officer, advised McGann that the school would be moved from Toronto to Hamilton. With this arbitrary notification, McGann contacted his pupils' families to ensure the students would report to Hamilton by rail and steamer that autumn.

In 1867, the school was moved to Dundurn Castle in Hamilton, but soon news came that the castle was to be sold, and once again the students were relocated, this time to premises on Main Street, where they remained until 1870.

It is interesting to note the comments of Rev. Dr. Egerton Ryerson in his 1868 report to the Ontario Legislature, saying that the instruction and training of two groups with such dramatically different sensory impairments would demand rather unique approaches. In this report, Dr. Ryerson's comments on blindness are revealing:

> ... if in the dark he is sometimes a king, in the light he is to be pitied and spared. But in the social circle, in the marts of trade, in the public hall, in the church — wherever speech of man flashes from mind to mind — he is at home. And his intellect ripening in the full sunshine, he often reaches the highest walks of eloquence, of poetry, and of philosophy. By universal consent, the blind Homer has sat for thousands of years in the highest seat of the temple of fame; and in later times few or none have climbed nearer his throne than the blind Milton.

What ought not to be missed or minimized in the conclusion of this cornerstone report is the clear acknowledgement that blindness incurs special costs and requires unique and specialized resources. From here onward, governments were reminded of this fact as a matter of public policy and social obligation:

> ... from the comparative helplessness of the Blind, and the kind of apparatus, instruments and books for their instruction in the ordinary elementary subjects, as well as in music, the education of the Blind is proportionally more expensive than that of the Deaf and Dumb, though suitable teachers for the Blind can be more easily obtained, and premises for their accommodation may be less extensive than for the Deaf and Dumb.

Ryerson then presented a detailed rationale that would lead to the creation, by 1870, of separate educational institutions for students who were blind and for those who were deaf.

McGann, like Ryerson, had reached the conclusion that a separate institution for the blind would be preferable. He offered $200 as a subscription toward opening an industrial establishment in Hamilton where blind people could learn trades. However, his idea was dropped when his school for the deaf was relocated to Belleville, where it continues today as the Sir James Whitney School for the Deaf, and the government decided to establish the Ontario Institution for the Blind in Brantford.

McGann died in 1880 and is buried in a Belleville cemetery. His students dedicated a memorial with the following inscription:

Sacred
to the memory of
John B. McGann,
Pioneer of Deaf-Mute Education
in Canada
Died
January 22nd, 1880
in his 69th year

Erected by the Deaf and Dumb of
Ontario, Canada

Although not mentioned in this inscription, his blind students have added their silent voice in tribute.

THE ONTARIO INSTITUTION FOR THE BLIND

While McGann was busy with his private school, a rather intriguing series of events was unfolding in the late 1860s within the halls of the Ontario provincial legislature. Attempts were being made to locate and establish a school for the blind, and a provisional committee, followed by a board of commissioners, was named by the minister of education to seek a suitable location.

After listening to presentations from various groups, the commissioners decided that Toronto or Hamilton would be most suitable. These cities, the commissioners reasoned, had good rail and water transport facilities, easy access to industrial markets for employing blind people and marketing the crafts and goods they produced, and exposure to first-class musicians who could motivate, inspire, and instruct blind musicians.

But because it was common practice for governments to decentralize major services and programs within various geographic areas of the country or province, even back then, it is not surprising that in 1872, the Ontario Institution for the Blind opened its doors to the first blind pupils in the town of Brantford, Ontario, twenty miles west of Hamilton and eighty-five miles west of Toronto.

When Brantford was chosen, the government of the day ignored the advice offered by Samuel G. Howe, the distinguished founder and principal of the Perkins Institution and Massachusetts Asylum for the Blind in Boston, Massachusetts, in a letter dated March 9, 1870:

> Bear in mind that one-half of your pupils will attempt to get a livelihood by teaching music, and that in order to become a good teacher of music, one must live in a musical atmosphere — must hear habitually the best music, and associate freely with the best performers. He cannot learn from precept or from teaching; he must hear habitually all the best musicians; and you may as well try to make sailors in an inland town as musicians in a village …

A second opinion, offered in a letter of March 11, 1870, to the Institution for the Deaf and Dumb and the Blind in Flint, Michigan, is direct and to the point: "… if you locate in a little, one-horse town, you will have a little, one-horse institution …"

In truth, and in vindication of Brantford, no evidence would suggest the decision to have been ill advised. In the end, what mattered was that at long last the blind youth and adults of Ontario were guaranteed education and training.

Operated and funded by the provincial government under the statutory provisions for asylums and prisons, this new school was named the Ontario Institution for the Blind. While in Nova Scotia the government opted to appoint a board of managers to oversee the Halifax school, in Ontario the Department of Education retained direct responsibility, an approach that later proved problematic.

The Ontario Institution for the Blind was later renamed the Ontario School for the Blind, and in 1974, the government of Ontario again renamed the school, this time as the W. Ross Macdonald School for the Blind in honour of a former provincial lieu-tenant-governor.

If renaming the school was even necessary, it would have been an excellent opportunity to recog-nize a prominent blind person, such as a former student. And what's more, throughout its long history, the school has never had a blind superintendent or principal.

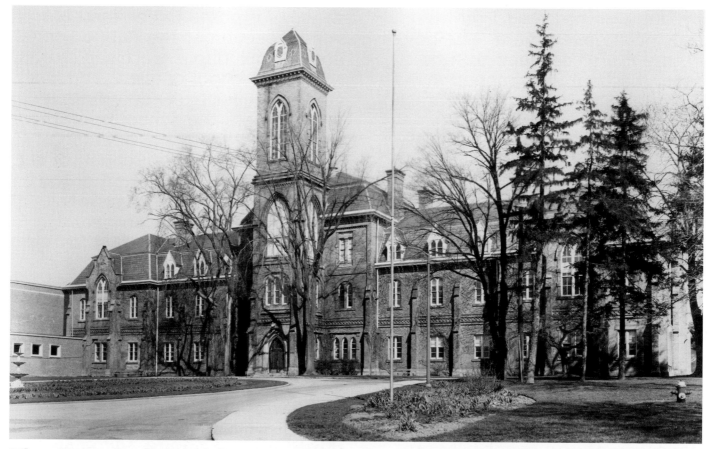

The Ontario School for the Blind, Brantford, Ontario, built in 1872.

BRITISH COLUMBIA: CANADA'S THIRD PROVINCIAL SCHOOL FOR THE BLIND

The first school for visually impaired children in British Columbia was the privately run School for Deaf-Mutes and the Blind, which opened in Victoria in September 1888. The school closed a year later after the founder, John Ashcroft, failed to secure a grant-in-aid from the provincial government. The government also declined to fund a second school that opened in Victoria in 1900, despite representations made by Victoria City Council and the British Columbia Benevolent Society. Beginning in 1901, however, the government provided grants for B.C. children attending approved schools for the deaf and blind outside the province. Most of the children were sent to the Manitoba School for the Deaf in Winnipeg.

By 1915, private citizens intervened when the provincial government, which had set as a priority the education of deaf children, was unreceptive to the idea of a specialized school for the blind. The government was eventually prevailed upon to accept the education of the blind as a public responsibility, but for financial expedience, and perhaps influenced by similar approaches in other countries, it undertook to educate deaf and blind children together.

In 1916, two blind people, A.A. Archibald and Mrs. C.E. Burke, organized British Columbia's first school for the blind in Burke's Vancouver home under the control and inspection of the Public School Board. Four pupils were registered when the school opened, and the number never exceeded ten over the six years the school operated.

By 1922, with the opening of the British Columbia School for the Deaf and Blind, education of the blind was assured. The school remained at its location near Jericho Beach in Vancouver's exclusive suburb of Point Grey throughout its history, with the exception of a temporary relocation to Burnaby during the Second World War.

The internment of Japanese-Canadians by the federal government was far-reaching and thorough, as described in *Moments in the History of Jericho Hill School,*

1915–1967 by Dr. Charles E. MacDonald, who was superintendent-principal of the school from 1934 to his retirement in 1967:

It was not long after the outbreak of World War II that all people of Japanese descent were moved away from the coastal areas of the Province. This wartime measure applied to half a dozen or so of our pupils. We were sorry, but could do nothing about it. Soon after the war ended, however, a request was granted to have Roi Matsune back in school. He was, I believe, one of the first of the Japanese to return to the Coast from the Interior. We were pleased to have him back, and he worked very hard to make up for lost time, as I recall. Most of the other pupils of Japanese origin had moved out of the Province or for some other reason did not return here.

The school was renamed Jericho Hill School in 1955, and for many years it enjoyed a good reputation, locally and nationally. But in the late 1970s and early 1980s, disquieting stories began circulating about instances of abuse at the school. Students who were known abusers were removed, although no charges were filed. But in 1991 a Vancouver newspaper published stories about rampant abuse at Jericho Hill, a public outcry followed, and in 1992 the provincial government closed the school. In 2004, a $12.5-million settlement with the provincial government was announced in a class-action lawsuit, which grew to include 350 people who were sexually abused at the school.

Although educators believed that children who are deaf have different needs from children who are blind, and educating them together is not in the best interests of either, the Jericho Hill School served both groups throughout its history.

EDUCATION IN THE PRAIRIE PROVINCES

In the nineteenth century, much of central western Canada formed part of a massive geographic area identified as the Northwest Territories. The population on the Prairies, with the exception of the Red River settlement at Winnipeg, was scattered and diverse, much as it is in the far north that comprises one-third of Canada's land mass. Manitoba attained provincial status within Confederation in 1870, while Saskatchewan and Alberta remained as a territory until 1905 when they, too, joined Confederation as the eighth and ninth provinces. A school for the blind in any of these provinces would have made little economic sense because there were relatively few eligible students.

For most of the twentieth century until the mid-1970s, the governments of Alberta, Saskatchewan, and Manitoba contracted with Ontario for blind students to attend the Ontario School for the Blind. Generations of blind students, aged six years and up, boarded Pullman sleeping cars in September, one for each Prairie province, and were transported to the school at Brantford for ten months until their return the following June.

For a short time prior to the closing of the Jericho Hill School, a small number of Alberta students attended that school as well.

From 1931 to 1948, Manitoba's Department of Education contracted to operate a small school for the blind on premises owned by the Canadian National Institute for the Blind on Portage Avenue that was, essentially, a single classroom. This fell outside of the CNIB charter and was in contravention of its stated policy not to engage in the direct education of young blind people.

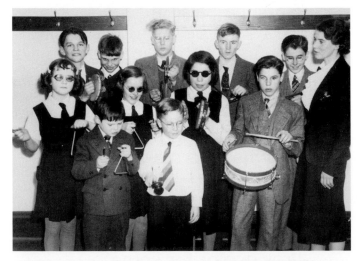

Blind and visually impaired children at the Manitoba School for the Blind, 1942.

EDUCATION AND THE OTHER PROVINCES

The governments in the other provinces where schools for the blind were never established recognized their responsibility toward blind youth and adopted the political and economic expedient of contracting out with the governments that operated these schools. Early on, New Brunswick and Prince Edward Island allocated funds to have the blind youth of their provinces educated in Halifax. It is rather interesting that colonial Newfoundland adopted this practice in the late nineteenth century and continued to do so after 1949 when it joined Confederation.

CLOSING OBSERVATIONS

Organized education for blind youth in Canada began around the late 1860s and continued for well over a century. The provincial schools in Halifax and Brantford and L'Institut Nazareth in Montreal extended their terms of reference and mandates to educate and train young adult blind Canadians. This

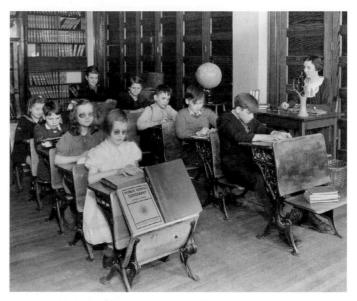

Blind pupils learn braille, 1936.

was done on a very limited basis but in direct response to the stark recognition that when a blind teenager had completed his formal education, access to advanced education, specialized training, and gainful employment would not be open to him. Blind students at these three schools who were fortunate enough to become accomplished musicians or to have acquired manual trades such as basketry, broom production, chair caning, and leather work were among Canada's first rehabilitated blind adults. Unfortunately, they were the exceptions, as most blind adults would be denied higher edu-

41

cation and gainful employment until well into the twentieth century.

The patchwork approach to the education of blind Canadians is, as mentioned earlier, mostly attributable to the nature of the Canadian federation. Although Canadian blind students were eventually integrated into mainstream education, the early years were a time of confusion and discrimination. By the late 1990s, there remained only one residential school for the blind in Canada — the school at Brantford, serving deaf-blind and multi-disabled blind students.

Today, throughout most of the world, blind children remain segregated for their education, with mainstreaming an emerging trend.

What the fragmented approach to educating blind children in the nineteenth and early part of the twentieth century really showed was that there was no strong federal organization for blind people that could coordinate services and speak for them.

CHAPTER 2
The CNIB Founders

The 1918 letters patent, or charter, for the Canadian National Institute for the Blind lists seven Canadians as signatories to its application for incorporation. All were men, five of them blind. Knowing this, however, is just the beginning, and inspires intriguing questions: Who were these individuals? What was their relationship with one another? Why were there seven? What motivated them? What inspired their vision for a national organization?

Answers to these and other questions are not easy to come by, as nearly a full century has passed from the planting of the early seeds of this national organization. With the exception of the biography of Edwin A. Baker, *No Compromise*, by Marjorie Wilkens Campbell, there is little information concerning the founders.

Before these seven men are introduced though, it's important to present other leading Canadians who may be considered founders as well. These individuals played a large part in heightening public awareness and helped to set the stage for the events of 1918 and what followed.

SIR CHARLES FREDERICK FRASER

Sir Charles Frederick Fraser must be counted as one of the earliest pioneers in work for the blind in Canada, with his contributions dating back to about 1873. One of fifteen children of a Nova Scotia physician, Fraser was injured at the age of about seven while whittling a stick with his new penknife. The eye became inflamed, his eyesight worsened, and by the time he was fourteen, he was blind. He graduated from the Perkins Institute for the Blind at the age of twenty-two and joined the Asylum for the Blind in Halifax as superintendent/teacher in 1873, a position he held for fifty years. His sphere of influence spread far beyond the school, and, judging from his persistent appeals to the government, he was undoubtedly a strong personality. His voice was heard in Ottawa and elsewhere,

and he was knighted in 1914. In 1977 the school was renamed Sir Frederick Fraser School, the only school for the blind in Canada to be named in honour of a blind educator.

Fraser's support for the founding of the Canadian National Institute for the Blind was sought because he had influence and prominence. Fraser, however, like others, was not convinced that a national organization to serve the blind was necessary, nor that it could succeed. A rather terse letter from Sherman Swift (one of the seven founders) dated October 3, 1917, to Sir Arthur Pearson, founder of St Dunstan's in England, a rehabilitation home for war-blinded servicemen, reads in part:

> ... now a word for your private ear ... unfortunately Canada, is like a house divided against itself, one association regarding with suspicion all others operating nearby or remotely in the district regarded as private preserves. It was thought advisable

by our Committee to prevent a possibility of opposition to the incorporation of the Institute by securing beforehand the support of several prominent blind Canadians. Foremost among these was Sir Frederick to secure his signature to the petition to Parliament. Now Sir Frederick is a man of considerable ability and one who has done great good to the blind of our Maritime Provinces. But his views of organization and development are limited very largely by the boundaries of his own limited geographical district. He is an autocrat and can therefore not brook the idea of anyone else sharing his power. The result of all this is that he has delayed, procrastinated, temporized and dragged out proceedings, objecting to this and that clause, inserting this and that word, protest-

ing against the invasion of what he calls "provincial" rights — and all the while taking the large national views of our own Committee, which he is, by underhand methods, attempting to turn to his own private and selfish advantage.

Swift goes on for three more pages in this vein and alleges that Fraser was attempting to establish a "Canadian St Dunstan's" in Halifax. His concluding request to Pearson is to "assist us to defeat his evident intentions re the National Institute by writing us some word of commendation of our movement."

As Fraser did not campaign publicly in opposition to the CNIB's formation, Swift's letter may not have been entirely fair, and when the CNIB established its Maritime division in 1919, Fraser, while declining the role of superintendent of the division, was, in the end, cooperative.

THE MONTREAL ASSOCIATION FOR THE BLIND

Two blind individuals in Montreal were also key players in the development of a national organization for the blind. Philip Layton, a blind piano tuner, arrived in Montreal from England in 1885. A successful businessman, he is credited with having founded the Montreal Association for the Blind (MAB) in 1909 and the Canadian Federation of the Blind (CFOB) in 1926. The MAB, approaching its centenary, is, in every respect, a successful service organization. Throughout its history it has operated workshops, maintained a school, provided a residence for the elderly blind, set up a modest library, and offered rehabilitation programs. The CFOB was a national consumer organization of blind people that ceased to exist in the mid-1950s.

Layton opposed the CNIB's formation as a national service organization. Although he joined forces with the CNIB on such important matters as a national pension for the blind, he was often said to be cantankerous and troublesome. Strained relationships from these early days persisted to

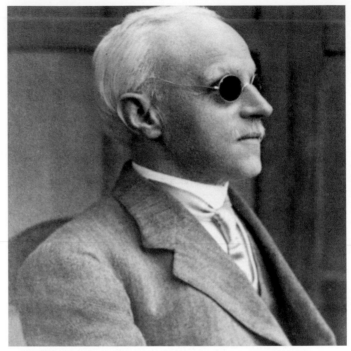

Philip Layton, founder of the Montreal Association for the Blind.

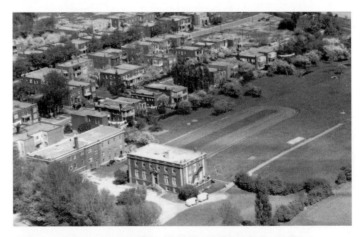

The Montreal Association for the Blind occupied prime real estate.

at least 1924, as seen in a letter dated October 12, 1925, from Lieutenant-Colonel Edwin Baker (another founding member of the CNIB) to Mr. Bedbrook of the MAB:

...we appreciate your desire for co-operation and would assure you that there can be nothing lacking on our part in this regard. You refer further to adhering to Ontario while you operate in Quebec province. You of course are aware that the Institute operates under a federal charter. We have endeavoured to keep clear of establishing any service in Quebec province which may have been previously organized and serving the needs of those concerned ... and ... with regard to our organization a biased critic has remarked "too many eggs in one basket." We have, however, preserved the equilibrium of the basket by close

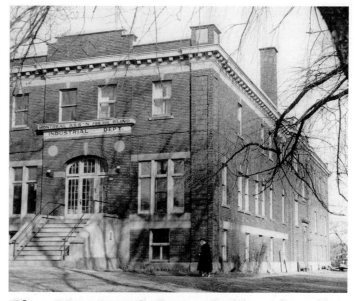

The Montreal Association for the Blind's industrial department.

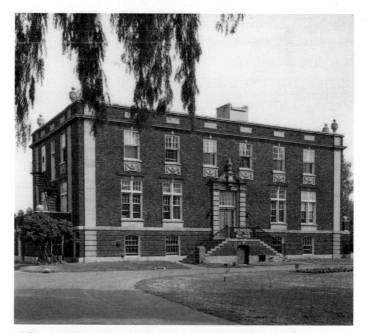

The Montreal Association for the Blind operated a school.

attention to the rights and privileges of each, and trust that we may never be found wanting in this regard.

Since both the MAB and the CNIB continue to flourish, whatever disagreement Layton and Baker may have had is now a curiosity of history.

Charles Lindsay, later to receive a knighthood, was another very successful blind businessman from England whose company became well known with the marketing of the Lindsay Piano. Like Layton, he was a piano tuner who immigrated to Montreal. Although he and Layton collaborated in the formation of the MAB, in Baker's view, Lindsay actually played the leading role. Regardless of who occupied the dominant position, these two individuals were well respected and deserve much credit for founding Canada's first rehabilitation agency for the blind. Lindsay went on to become a volunteer with the CNIB in Quebec and was instrumental in the formation of a CNIB division in that province in 1930.

SANDFORD LEPPARD

Although Sandford Leppard was not a signatory to the CNIB charter, he played an active role throughout his long life in the CNIB's development. In 1957, at the age of ninety-five, he was presented to Queen Elizabeth II on her visit to the CNIB's Fragrant Garden on the Bayview Avenue campus, where he was introduced as Canada's oldest living blind citizen. He corrected Ralph Misener, CNIB's national president at the time, and informed Her Majesty that there was a blind woman in attendance who was, in fact, one hundred. A clipping from a 1958 newspaper article entitled, "OSB's Oldest 'Old Boy' Returns for Ceremonies" reveals details of his career and contribution:

The oldest "Old Boy" of them all returned to the Ontario School for the Blind last night. Sandford Leppard of Toronto … is the only surviving member of the original class at the school in 1872. Mr. Leppard was born near

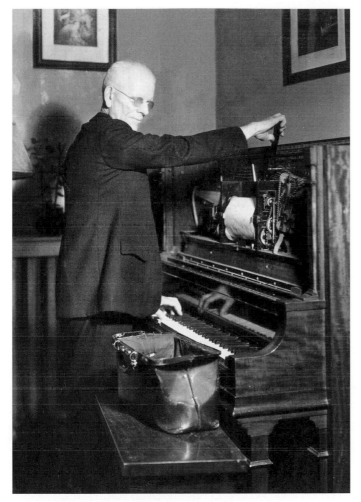

Sandford Leppard was an accomplished piano tuner.

vice-president of the CNIB and vice-chairman of the Ontario Division.

HARRIS TURNER

Harris Turner, a First World War blinded veteran, served in the Saskatchewan provincial legislature and was a successful publisher, founding the *Western Producer* newspaper and other publications.

Baker thought a great deal of Turner's ability, and after Turner retired to the West Coast, Baker persuaded him to work for the CNIB in Toronto in national public relations, which he did for ten years.

SIR WILLIAM MULOCK

Newmarket, Ontario, learned the theory of piano tuning at the OSB and started his own business in 1925. Mr. Leppard is a life member of the CNIB. He is senior

Sir William Mulock, who was Canada's postmaster general in 1898, made enormous contributions to the blind. He is credited with making Canada one of the first countries, if not the first country, in the world to adopt franking legislation that permitted postal delivery of embossed materials for blind people and schools for the blind free of charge. An excerpt from *Hansard*, dated April 1, 1898, gives an account of at least two advocates who sought this exemption:

> … The Postmaster General [Mulock] moved for leave to introduce Bill [No. 110] to amend the Post Office Act.
>
> and
>
> … That suggestion has been made to me by Mr. C.F. Fraser of Halifax, who, I understand, is connected with an institute for the blind and the subject has also been pressed upon me by Mr. Dymond, who is the superintendent of the Blind Asylum in Brantford.

Mulock's actions soon led to an expanded circulation of embossed books, first from the schools for the blind and then, after 1906, from the Free Library for the Blind in Toronto. For nearly one hundred years, this priceless legislation has not only served blind Canadians through the CNIB's lending library but has gone on to become a worldwide movement. Today, 180 of the 189 member countries of the Universal Postal Union, the global postal network that regulates the international exchange of mail, deliver materials — printed matter, audio books, video cassettes, and CDs — for the blind at no cost.

EDGAR ROBINSON

Edgar Bertram Freel Robinson was part of a select group whose members were able to pursue a university education at a time when this was almost unthinkable. Born in Stouffville, Ontario, in 1872, Robinson attended the Ontario School for the Blind. In 1893 he graduated from Trinity College in Toronto with the designation of Philosophy Prizeman for that year.

His book, *The True Sphere of the Blind*, published by William Briggs in 1896, is an interesting thesis on the psychological aspects of blindness. Robinson's academic achievements are remarkable for the day, and his work is the first Canadian publication by a blind author on the subject of blindness.

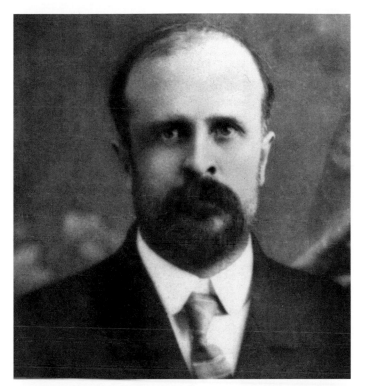

Edgar Bertram Freel Robinson, founder of the Free Library for the Blind.

... the number of volumes loaned has surpassed the most sanguine expectations of the most enthusiastic of our members. It was thought that many would have to be induced to take to reading and that our work should for a time be considered as educative largely, but nothing of the kind proved necessary as within a very few weeks after opening we found that we could not supply the demand, especially the demand for those books which we have ourselves had embossed.

Eager to share his private collection of braille books with other blind readers, in 1906 he founded the Free Library for the Blind from his small home in Markham, Ontario. As will soon be evident, the board members of this library were to play a key role in the CNIB's incorporation. At the second annual meeting of the library in February 1908, Robinson was able to report:

Sadly, Robinson died suddenly of typhoid on November 7 of that same year; he was only thirty-six. Had he lived, it is entirely possible he would have been one of the founders of the CNIB.

SIR ARTHUR PEARSON

Sir Arthur Pearson, who founded St Dunstan's in England in 1915, is

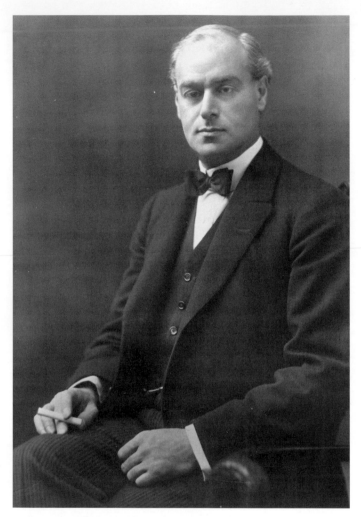

Sir Arthur Pearson.

hand in the formation of the CNIB and served as the new organization's first honorary president.

His friendship and influence with several of the founders of the CNIB placed him in the role of mentor and confidant. He knew Edwin Baker and Alexander Viets, two of the seven founders, from their rehabilitation at St Dunstan's in London; evidently the three spent a good deal of time together at social events. Baker, when asked later in life whom he considered to be the largest world personage he had met during his career, replied that Arthur Pearson had influenced him and impressed him the most.

THE WOMEN'S ASSOCIATION FOR THE WELFARE OF THE BLIND

prominent among visionaries in the rehabilitation of the blind. From its inception to the present day, St Dunstan's has served war-blinded and blind veterans and their families; Canadians blinded in both world wars received rehabilitation there. Pearson had a direct

Men, most of them blind, weren't the only ones who had come together to shape a national blindness service organization; the presence and influence of prominent women well predates the 1918 charter. The Women's Association for the Welfare of the Blind (WAWB) was established to assist the Canadian Free Library for the Blind, which, by 1917, had changed its name to the Canadian National Library for the Blind.

Mrs. W.A.H. Kerr, president of the WAWB, had a personal interest because she was the cousin of Dr. Charles Dickson, a founder.

Mrs. Lionel Clarke, the wife of the lieutenant-governor of Ontario, led a corps of volunteer women in Toronto who not only provided support services to blind people but also, far more importantly, gave financial stability to two struggling organizations, namely the Free Library for the Blind and the CNIB.

There is no explanation to be had as to why the people mentioned here, and others, are not recognized as charter members of the CNIB. Whatever the reason may be for this lack of recognition, the contributions of these individuals are certainly in evidence.

THE GROUP OF SEVEN

Now, having paid tribute to these leading individuals, it is time to meet the seven men who are recognized as charter members of the Canadian National Institute for the Blind:

AND WHEREAS LEWIS MILLER WOOD, Financial Agent; SHERMAN CHARLES SWIFT, Librarian; ALEXANDER GRISWOLD VIETS, Insurance Agent; EDWIN ALBERT BAKER, Electrical Engineer; CHARLES REA DICKSON, Physician; GEORGE GORDON PLAXTON, and CHARLES WATTY CARRUTHERS, Barristers, all of the City of Toronto, in the Province of Ontario, have made application for a charter under the said Act, constituting them and such others as may become members in the corporation thereby created a body corporate and politic, under the name of THE CANADIAN NATIONAL INSTITUTE FOR THE BLIND.

There is no real explanation why the men's names appear in the order they do on the letters patent. The names are not alphabetical, and Lewis Wood was not the founding president, although his name appears first. Be that as it may, they will be introduced in this chapter with the five men who were blind discussed first, then the two who were sighted.

Among the group of five blind men, there was a deep, underlying friendship.

ALEXANDER VIETS

Alexander Griswold Viets was born in Digby, Nova Scotia, in 1878 and enlisted in the army in Calgary in 1914. Blinded by a mortar explosion in France early in the First World War, he was sent to St Dunstan's for rehabilitation, where he shared a room with Edwin Baker and Clutha MacKenzie, who went on to become well-known for his work with the blind in New Zealand and Asia. It's easy to imagine these young, smart, newly blinded men discussing their thoughts on the rehabilitation of the blind, given their proximity to the National Institute for the Blind in London and the programs offered at St Dunstan's.

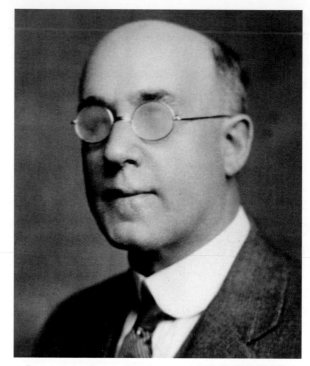

Alexander Griswold Viets.

Viets was the first soldier blinded in the First World War to return to Canada from St Dunstan's. Although he went home to Nova Scotia, he was encouraged by Baker to move to Toronto, where he was employed by the Imperial Life Assurance Company of Canada in 1916; he joined the board of the Canadian National Library for the Blind later that year. He served as a vice-president of the CNIB and was awarded the King's Medal in 1937. Viets was described as a thoughtful and quiet contributor to the new organization with a good head for business. He died at the age of seventy-one.

EDWIN BAKER

It is neither prudent nor necessary to attempt to expand on Lieutenant-Colonel Edwin Albert Baker's life and role with the work of the CNIB beyond that which is contained in his published biography. However, no account of his involvement with the CNIB can ever do justice to the enormity of his vision, influence, and reach. A single-minded tactician, he was energetic, charming, and handsome with an extraordinary talent for attracting and influencing those around him.

Born near Kingston, Ontario, in 1893, Baker was a graduate of Queen's University's engineering program. Blinded by a sniper's bullet in Belgium in 1915, Baker underwent a period of rehabilitation at St Dunstan's, returned to Toronto in 1916, and was immediately appointed to the board of the Free Library for the Blind. Soon after, he was hired by Sir Adam Beck at the Ontario Hydro Electric

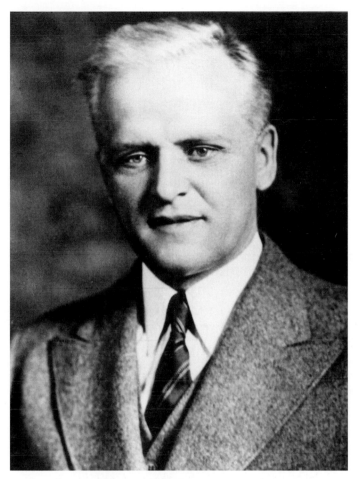

Edwin Albert Baker.

Power Commission and worked there from October of that year until he was recruited by the federal government as a consultant on services to the war-blinded in 1918. From that distance, Baker participated in the founding of the CNIB, was appointed its first vice-president in 1918, and in 1920 returned to Toronto to accept paid employment with the CNIB as its second managing director, a position he held for forty-two years until his retirement in 1962. He died in April 1968.

Baker's influence and pioneering nature led not only to the founding of the CNIB but also to the founding of other national and international organizations in the field of blindness and blindness prevention. Employees and acquaintances alike speak of him with glowing respect and admiration. His eldest son, John, at his 1987 retirement as president of the CNIB's National Council, presented Baker's military and civil medals of honour at the annual general meeting. These seven medals are proudly displayed in the CNIB's national boardroom and are a concise and powerful biography of a patriotic man's life and career.

Sherman Charles Swift.

SHERMAN SWIFT

Sherman Charles Swift was born in 1879 in Petrolia, Ontario, and lost his sight as a young boy in a gunpowder explosion. He attended the Ontario School for the Blind at Brantford and earned an Honours B.A. from McGill University in 1907, majoring in modern languages. At the Ontario School for the Blind he became friends with

Charles Carruthers, and later the two men became friends with E.B.F. Robinson. After Robinson's untimely death in 1908, his wife carried on his work until 1911, when Swift was appointed Librarian of the Free Library for the Blind. Charles Carruthers and Charles Dickson, who also served as board members, joined him in this work.

Swift earned a master's degree from the Faculty of Education at the University of Toronto. He spoke seven languages fluently and in 1908 was the first qualified blind person to apply for teaching certification — he was refused, but certification was granted fifteen years later.

He was the author of many unpublished poems and co-author of *The Voyages of Jacques Cartier in Prose and Verse* (1934). As a founder, he proved to be a force to be reckoned with.

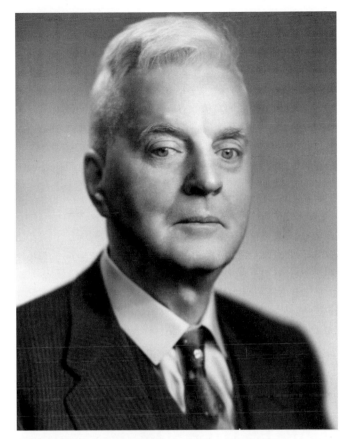

Charles Watty Carruthers.

CHARLES CARRUTHERS

Dr. Charles Watty Carruthers was born in Avening, Ontario, in 1886 and lost his sight at age five through an undiagnosed illness.

He attended the Ontario School for the Blind from age five to fourteen, and then Woodstock College, Pickering College, and the University of Toronto, where he earned a B.A. He went on to qualify for admission to the Bar at Osgoode Hall, but, possibly finding it difficult to establish a law practice, he became interested in osteopathy and attended a school of osteopathy in Des Moines, Iowa. He interned in Missouri and returned to Toronto, where he set up a practice at Danforth and Carlaw avenues that lasted forty years. Carruthers taught braille to blinded First World War veterans and was president of the Canadian National Library for the Blind at the time of its amalgamation with the CNIB National Library. He was awarded the Canadian Centennial Medal in 1967 and was a president of the International Association of Blind Osteopaths. He was the last surviving founder and died at the age of ninety in 1976.

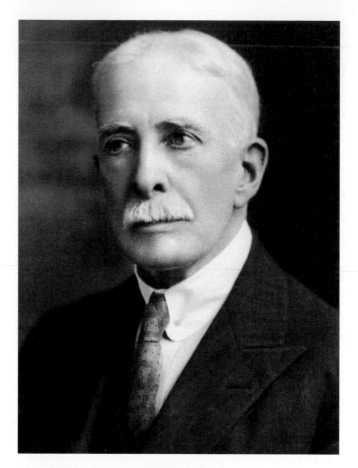

Charles Rae Dickson.

CHARLES DICKSON

Dr. Charles Rae Dickson, born in Kingston, Ontario, in 1858, was considerably older than the other six founders. A graduate of Queen's University, he had an illustrious medical career as a pioneer in X-ray technology and was head of that department at Toronto General Hospital. It was reported that Dr. Dickson was blinded in 1908 at age fifty when an early X-ray experiment went wrong. He served as the first president of the CNIB, was awarded the King's Medal, and was made a Knight of the Order of St. John of Jerusalem for founding the Canadian branch of the St. John's Ambulance. He died in 1938 while serving as vice-president of the CNIB.

GEORGE PLAXTON AND LEWIS WOOD

The final two players associated with the Library's operations were two sighted men, George Gordon Plaxton, who served as honorary solicitor, and Lewis Miller Wood. On a pro bono basis, Plaxton crafted the CNIB's articles of incorporation. Within a year or so of incorporation, he returned to his law practice, maintaining only a limited association with the new national agency.

Lewis Wood, a Halifax native who lived in New York for a period of time, moved to Toronto in the early 1900s. He and his brother constructed the original Royal Bank Building in downtown Toronto, one of the first skyscrapers erected in Canada. Wood met Baker at the home of John Robinson, publisher of the *Toronto Telegram*, and at this first meeting, it is reported that Wood had not realized that Baker was blind and asked his host, Robinson, why Baker had left without saying good evening. Upon hearing the explanation, he became intrigued and wanted to meet Baker again. From this beginning, the two become lifelong friends.

When the Free Library for the Blind fell on hard times and was given notice to vacate the room it occupied in the basement of a west Toronto library building, Baker contacted Wood to see if he could help obtain financial assistance. At a meeting in January 1917, when Baker proposed that

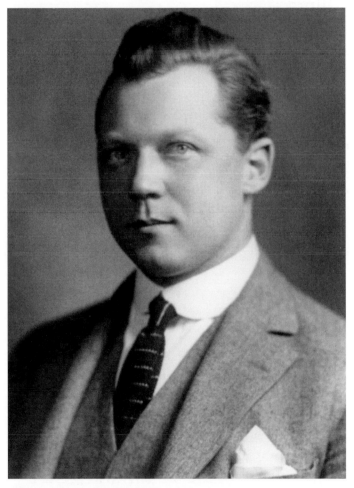

George Gordon Plaxton.

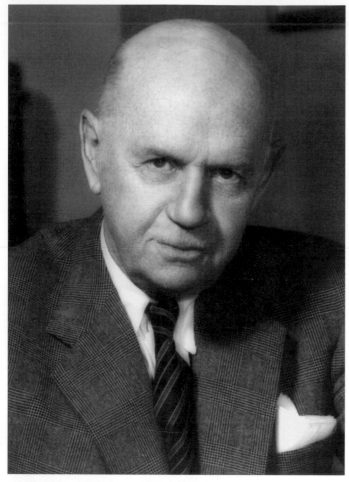

Lewis Miller Wood.

Wood be invited to head a finance committee, a board member opposed the recruiting of a sighted person. Baker replied that Wood's credibility and influence would prove invaluable in soliciting large donations and would reassure a sighted business community that the funds were carefully accounted for. In Baker's words, "the sighted world does not believe that blind people can adequately manage large funds ... they don't today, but someday they will."

Wood not only bailed out the Free Library for the Blind by obtaining donations from his wide circle of business acquaintances, he continued to raise funds throughout his association with the CNIB. In the early years, when the fledgling organization was desperately short of cash, Wood would head out to a golf course or a club and return to the CNIB with a cheque for the required funds.

As president of National Council for thirty-four years, from 1918 to 1952, Wood was a powerful, if quiet, influence on the CNIB's founding. Although he went on to play a leadership role in the formation of other national charitable organizations, his leadership as the senior volunteer for the CNIB is a remarkable record of achievement. He was both a confidant and mentor to Baker, and the two regularly travelled to Ottawa and other parts of Canada on institute business.

THE GROUP IN ACTION

Whether through friendship or professional association, this group of seven had come together, and by 1918 all were well acquainted and residing in Toronto.

A little before this, though, in the spring of 1917, discussion at the Canadian National Library for the Blind Board had focused on the need for a more generalized national organization to serve the blind in Canada. It was at this point that the work to draft the articles of incorporation began in earnest.

The five blind founders spent a good deal of time at Dr. Dickson's house at 192 Bloor Street in Toronto. With the group gathered around his kitchen table, the atmosphere and conversation would have been elevating and stimulating. All these men held strong views and were passionate on matters of politics and the rights of blind people, not only to shape and control their own destiny but also to speak for themselves and to be heard. Several excerpts from exchanges of correspondence reveal much about the personalities and thoughts of these individuals.

Consider this letter of October 16, 1916, from Swift to Dickson, referring to the Ontario School for the Blind:

> … From the date of its foundation more than forty years ago the School has been made a juicy plum to be plucked and enjoyed by some henchman of the reigning political party, for whom a reward for faithful service had to be found. When the investigation, about which you know, was concluded recently, such a shocking condition of affairs in every department was laid bare that it was hoped our government would at last awaken to the fact of the viciousness of the system it had found in vogue when it came into power, but which it was short-sighted enough (not to say selfish enough) to perpetuate … The very class most in need of enlightened and

scientific training has been callously and contemptuously turned over to political henchmen, for whom something had to be done and whose duties as head of our School for the Blind were considered as sinecures...with proper training the blind are capable of mingling on equal terms with the most cultured of the nation — but such training our government has not only neglected to afford, it has refused to consider it ... We are no longer the timid and leaderless sheep we once were, but we have become conscious of ourselves and have measured our rights.

On August 18, 1916, Dickson wrote to Sir R.A. Pyne, the Ontario Minister of Education, who was in London, England, at the time, regarding the appointment of a new principal for the Ontario School for the Blind:

... you have a splendid opportunity to show what kind of stuff you are made of ... I implore you not to repeat that fool-trick of the Grits by placing in a position of such importance to those already terribly handicapped, a man whose only qualification is that he is a member of our own party. I am a Conservative from the crown of my head to the sole of my feet and I want my party to commit no such crime for it is nothing short of a crime to the Blind ...You will have a splendid opportunity while in England to go and see Sir Arthur Pearson. Ask him what he thinks about blind teachers for blind people. He can tell. Ask him about political heelers as principals. Then go and see some schools for the Blind and take notes. And when you come home be a civilized human being with a conscience, not a party hack!

Swift's insight and spirit as a fierce advocate for the blind is revealed in this letter to Wood, written on May 11, 1917:

> … the Canadian public is only beginning to wake up to the fact that Canada has a "blind question," and I fear our Federal authorities, like those of the provinces, will not be better informed than the voters. Some years ago the Dominion Government was approached with a view to securing a small grant. We were informed that such grant could not be given, since our work was a charity and that if we were assisted, other charities would claim equal right. I need not point out to you that the charity attitude of the public mind toward the blind is not only terribly wounding to the sensibilities of the intelligent sightless, being wholly unjustified by the facts, but it also prevents both government and public alike from attacking the problem in a spirit of enlightenment and sincere desire to assist. The blind do not ask for charity, but they do ask, and they have a right to ask, that they be given a chance to make good to the limits which their handicap sets to their powers.

Wood's reply the following day is reassuring to Swift, and in it, he also commits to being a key player for the organization:

> … I feel very strongly that I could assist you very much in the financial end of your work and would be very much obliged if I could have an opportunity of analyzing the financial con-

dition of your institution and of familiarizing myself with the ambitions and plans that you have for the future.

On September 8, 1916, Dickson wrote a lively letter to Viets, who was about to move to Toronto. He offered to help Viets find work and wrote of his vision for the future institute for the blind. The text of this letter reveals Dickson's thoughts a year before the CNIB's founding constitution was actually drafted.

... we will arm ourselves with Bowie knives and hold them at the throats of the men we interview and we will surely land something good for you. Of course we will not start that way, it would be neither necessary nor politic, but I know lots of people here and will do all I can for you most gladly ...
... had a nice telephone chat with Baker today. I may be able to help him with a sales-manship job, electrical machinery. He will be here some weeks. He wished to be remembered to you. I said I had heard from you today. I am corresponding with London re a Canadian National Institute for the Blind. London wants us to affiliate. Col. Chas. Hodgetts is conducting negotiations. Am corresponding with Sir F. Fraser on same lines ...
We want a Canadian National Institute badly and we want it NOW. So we are going to get it — soon. I am not paying any attention to obstacles but am starting with our Eastern Provinces and working Westward Ho! My plan is to have every legitimate activity for the Blind represented in this Institute. Each will be asked in turn. The Institute will be incorporated whether all come in or not, but we would prefer to have everyone

represented. We will have to get over petty jealousies and provincialism and all that tommy-rot if we ever expect to arrive anywhere and we are going to arrive. I will not burden you with the name of our chief obstacle specialist in case he or she repents later or and is very, very, sorry, etc. ...

Sir Frederick is in favour of work for the Blind and willing to help but is bothering his head about who should take the initiative. I would like to see him the Honorary President of the new body and have told him so. I want him to head the list of applicants for a charter but have not got to details yet with him, nor even the name of the new body ...

The idea is, not to interfere in the slightest way with any institution, but allow it to conduct its own affairs just as before, each one to be entirely independent of the other and of the C.N.I.B. The chief function of the latter will be to collect funds for all, supplementing present methods. As many organizations as possible will be interested in the work and assist in the collections, this will allow the various Field Secretaries to have more time for other pressing work in connection with their schools, etc. It will be on the lines of the British Institute as far as possible and for the good of the Blind of all Canada. One of the first things will be to initiate a publishing department for the reproduction of books not now available in Braille also text books. Gradually it will extend to other much needed activities not now existing here. It will strive to assist every legitimate activity now in operation and to establish others where needed. It will strive to secure work and situations for the Blind. It will endeavour to secure much needed legislation and the appointment of a Permanent Federal Commission on the Blind. Every activity will be represented on its Board of Management whatever name it chooses to call that Board. I hope to see you on that Board too.

A disquieting footnote to Dickson's brilliance and leadership are comments made about him by Charles W. Holmes, the CNIB's first director, on a History Sheet dated October 15, 1920:

> … owing both to his impracticability, lack of executive capacity and temperamental idiosyncrasies, Dr. Dickson unfortunately has stood very much in his own light as well as in the light of those things

which he has undertaken to further. He was replaced as President of the Institute in August 1918 and as General Secretary in January 1919 … Pearson Hall had just opened and he was placed in charge thereof. Another signal failure was made of his relation in this capacity and matters at the Hall got into such bad state and so far beyond control that in June 1919 he was replaced there and was retired upon an annuity to continue at the discretion of the Executive Committee with some nominal duties in the way of publicity …

This one man's view may have lacked objectivity, but it does report on significant events. Dickson's style and flamboyance contributed to the group's synergy and energy, which in the end accomplished their goal. Almost sixty when the CNIB was founded, with maturity and impressive network of contacts, he was an excellent role model for the other founders, who were mostly in their twenties.

No single one of these seven founders is credited above any other with having played a leading role during these formative years. Through personal friendships and mutual respect, supported by their unique backgrounds and shared values, each of these individuals helped bring into focus a vision of a national service organization. They withstood the criticisms and opposition of those who did not support or believe in the value and purpose of a national service organization. The objects for this organization, as set out in the charter, provided the breadth and scope of activities that could and would eventually be undertaken. Programs dealing with the welfare of the blind, their education and employment, libraries, and other cultural activities still remain provincial and municipal responsibilities.

But now there exists an organization embodied in one federal charter that, over time, has structured itself into ten operating divisions covering Canada's ten provinces and three territories. The CNIB stands unparalleled in rehabilitation and training in the field of Canadian disability.

If, from time to time, there were disputes among these founders or hesitation in moving forward with incorporation, those thoughts and discussions are not now known. The collective wisdom and energy of these seven men, and of the other men and women who aligned themselves with their cause, initiated a revolution in services to the blind that enlightened not only Canadian society but also the rest of the world.

CHAPTER 3
The Founders in Action

By 1918, Canadian forces had been fighting in the First World War for nearly four years. Most historians agree that it was during this watershed period, which included the decision by Parliament to raise and send an expeditionary force to the European theatre of war and the consequences that followed, that Canada came of age as a nation.

Canada's involvement in this war had a dramatic effect on the national psyche and helped raise awareness of political and social issues among Canadians. And as part of this new awareness, the incorporation of a new organization brought into sharp focus a disability group whose numbers may have been relatively small but whose needs were distinctive: people who had been blinded, whatever the cause of their loss of sight.

Two separate but related events would add considerable impetus, urgency, and energy to the CNIB's early years.

On the morning of December 6, 1917, *Mont Blanc*, a French munitions ship, collided with *Imo*, a Belgian relief vessel, and blew up in Halifax Harbour, causing one of the worst manmade disasters ever. About two thousand people were killed, and among the nine thousand injured survivors were almost forty — including several members of the same family — who had been permanently blinded in an instant from shooting shards of shattered glass. Hundreds more people were left visually impaired from their injuries. In her book *Shattered City: The Halifax Explosion and the Road to Recovery*, Janet Kitz writes that more than 1,000 eye cases were treated, with more than 250 eye removals performed over a period of about two weeks. In the end, thirty-seven people — eight men, twenty women, and nine children — were left sightless, although many of the dead had also been blinded. Two hundred and six survivors had lost one eye and needed monitoring to ensure that they retained their vision in the other. Two hundred and sixty more people had glass embedded in their eyes.

The small, closely knit Halifax community, supported by national and international efforts, rallied to provide medical care and housing for the wounded, and the Halifax School for the Blind provided ready resources and quickly accepted a number of individuals for rehabilitation.

Overseas, meanwhile, the war in Europe was taking an enormous toll on the small army of young Canadian soldiers. Thousands were killed in those foreign fields, and many more were left blinded from injuries sustained in battle, including the effects of shellfire, bombs, or mustard gas poisoning. Many war-blinded soldiers, of course, had also suffered other injuries, including loss of limbs and what was then called shell shock, now known as post-traumatic stress disorder.

Following medical treatment in the field or in hospitals in France or England, selected war-blinded soldiers, including E.A. Baker, the first Canadian officer to lose his sight in the war, were offered rehabilitation at St Dunstan's hostel. St Dunstan's was founded in 1915 by Sir Arthur Pearson, a wealthy English newspaper baron who had lost his sight to glaucoma in 1912. The mission behind St Dunstan's was revolutionary in its day: it was believed that with the

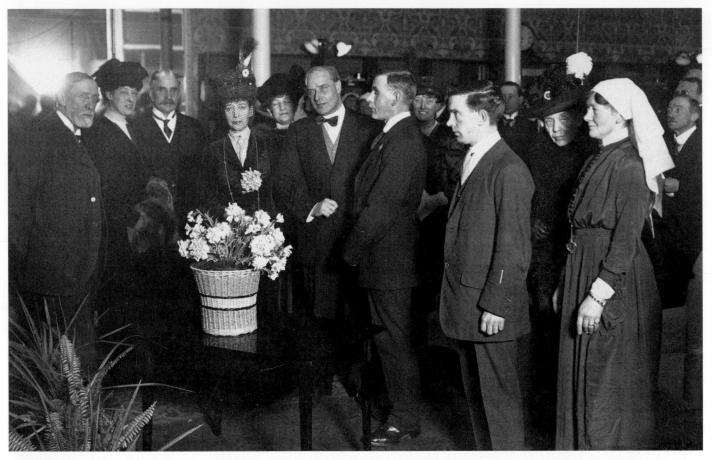

Queen Alexandra, behind a basket of carnations, visits St Dunstan's. On her right is Canadian Prime Minister Sir Robert Borden, and on her left is Sir Arthur Pearson.

right training, war-blinded soldiers and sailors could take their place in society as productive, contributing members and lead useful and satisfying lives.

Located in a large converted house near London's Regent's Park, St Dunstan's provided a pleasant and safe environment in which recently blinded servicemen could learn trades such as carpentry, shoe-making, basketry, or weaving, as well as life-enhancing skills such as braille and typing.

By May of 1918, the first thirty-one blind soldiers had been returned directly to Canada, where no suitable rehabilitation services existed for them. In June, all blind Canadian soldiers still in Europe were offered the opportunity to go to St Dunstan's, and the soldiers already repatriated to Canada were given the chance to return to England for rehabilitation.

Soldiers who had returned to Canada before 1918 without passing through the St Dunstan's program had three options open to them: to attend the Halifax School for the Blind as an adult, to obtain services from the Montreal Association for the Blind (which had been in operation since 1909), or to return home to their families and communities without having received any kind of training to prepare them to live out their lives as blind people.

The frustration and despondency of the situation in which these newly blinded men found themselves is captured in a heart-wrenching and eloquent letter written by thirty-three-year-old Abel Knight, a corporal in the Princess Patricia's Canadian Light Infantry. Knight, who was born in Manchester, England, enlisted in Calgary on August 8, 1914, and was wounded at Ypres in May 1915.

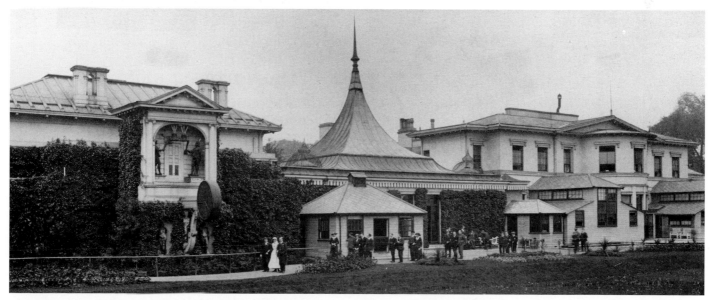

St Dunstan's, Regent's Park, London, England.

Writing from the Halifax School for the Blind on February 20, 1918, to Dr. Dickson in Toronto, Knight begins by thanking him politely for the braille watch "received today" and goes on to say:

> In your letter to Mr. McMillan you ask among other particulars what professions we intend to follow. Well, after six months at this Institute, I can only reply that, "I don't know." I came here last September, enthusiastic and under the impression that I should meet men who have studied the blind adult question. My experience here has proved to me beyond all doubt that having got us here the officials of this Institute considered their labours ended.
>
> Any complaint is met by the question, "What do you want to do?"
>
> I ask you, Sir, "If Sir Frederick Fraser, after 45 years experience among the blind, does not know what a blind adult can do, how the devil can I, who was blinded by misadventure in the Ypres Salient, be expected to know?
>
> When I came here I brought my wife and child in order that I might see them as long as possible. But patriotism in this city was of such a high order that although I advertised for rooms in the daily papers, as a blinded soldier, mark you, I received no replies. I suppose the little hearted inhabitants of this city thought a soldier at $1.10 per day hardly worthwhile. I finally got the use of three unheated rooms for which I paid $35 per month. My finances could not stand the strain and I sent my wife and child back to Alberta last month.
>
> I am now alone. Until last month there were no Braille writers that would write in this place.

I received my first lesson on a print typewriter two weeks ago, so am yet dependent on others to write my letters. True, a course of massage can be taken here, but I don't like that profession, nor am I prepared to become an itinerant vendor of scrubbing brushes.

The only thing achieved in my case here is the killing of all ambition due to the uncongenial surroundings, and of course any attempt at friendliness by the inhabitants now would, in view of their past indifference, be regarded with suspicion.

My only desire now is to get home to my family, re-education or no re-education.

Thanking you again, I am

Yours truly,
Abel Knight.

While in Halifax, Knight, who had survived the 1917 Halifax explosion, is credited with founding the Overseas Veterans League, which became the Royal Canadian Legion.

Unemployment and poverty were almost guaranteed for war-blinded servicemen without resources or independent means. Although well-intentioned community organizations such as women's groups or churches often assumed responsibility for the care of the indigent poor as charity cases and provided minimal food and shelter for them, many Canadians felt that the federal government had a moral responsibility to care for that special group of men who had been blinded in the service of their country. Unfortunately, a number of these men slipped through the cracks while jurisdictions argued over who should take care of them.

It was within this framework, then, that the founders of the CNIB pressed ahead to create a national organization that would provide service and speak for blind Canadians. Until now, the founders had focused on civilians and had been active in lobbying governments at all levels, as well as the public, for financial support.

THE NEW CNIB

Baker and Viets had returned from St Dunstan's in 1916. As blind veterans, they quickly turned to Ottawa to advocate on behalf of all war-blinded veterans, explaining that the choices were to have the blinded veterans return to England for training or to establish programs for them in Canada. While both approaches were adopted, the preference became to offer services in Toronto, where the new CNIB was headquartered.

The new CNIB, however, was struggling with other issues.

By the spring of 1917, the Canadian National Library for the Blind was in serious financial difficulty. Baker and Wood stabilized the library by leasing quarters at 142 College Street from the University of Toronto and obtaining working capital for its continued operation. The Toronto Women's Musical Club was also drawn in to provide furniture and secure financial support.

On March 30, 1918, at a meeting at which the seven founders were present, George Plaxton, a solicitor, presented a letter from the Canadian government's under-secretary of state informing him that letters patent, which formally incorporated the institute, had been issued. Bylaws were read and adopted as the first general bylaws of the new organization. With everything officially now in place, the founders moved to establish an effective, functioning service organization. From rented rooms at 36 King Street East, today the site of Canadian Press, they went into action.

Dickson was elected president, and Baker, who would devote the rest of his career to the CNIB, was made vice-president. Kathleen Junkin, who was soon joined by the young Grace Worts, provided secretarial support.

The new executive, known as National Council, decided that as a priority they should hire a director. After a brief search, and at the suggestion of librarian Sherman Swift, they interviewed and hired Charles W. Holmes, who had been born in Quebec, was a graduate of Boston's Perkins School for the Blind, and at the time of his hiring was superintendent of the Massachusetts Institute for the Blind. A former president of the American Association of Workers

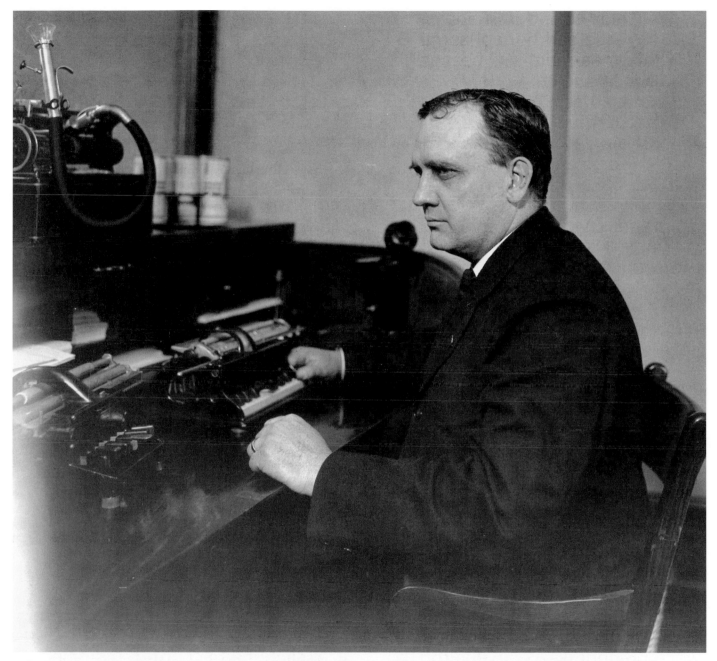

Charles W. Holmes, the CNIB's first director, in his office at 36 King Street East, Toronto, with brailling and dictating equipment.

for the Blind, Holmes was a violinist and organist and had studied music in Germany.

Holmes was given a five-year contract, to run from July 1, 1918, at a salary of $2,500 per year, with an annual increase of $100 per annum. However, in May 1919, his salary was increased to $3,000 per year.

Holmes's job description, although somewhat vague, was certainly demanding. His contract stipulates that he would be expected "to devote his whole time and energies to the furtherance of the objects of the Institute and to perform such duties as shall be assigned to him from time to time by the Council …" He was also expected to act quickly and decisively to launch various programs to enhance daily living, such as personal grooming. Courses and programs related to employment, such as typing, the reading and writing of braille, and vocational training, were larger goals and would take longer.

With hindsight, it becomes apparent that the CNIB was not so much "founded" as "evolved." It came into being as an outgrowth of already established organiza-tions and institutions such as schools for the blind. Many associations, however, were reluctant to give up their autonomy and refused to amalgamate or affiliate with the new broad-based organization. The Montreal Association for the Blind, some schools, and the Canadian National Library for the Blind were among those that distanced themselves and held on to their financial and human resources for their own programs.

Other organizations, like the National Council of Women of Canada, the Canadian Women's Association for the Welfare of the Blind, and the Ontario Association for the Blind, joined forces early on, and in June 1918, elected representatives from these organizations joined the CNIB's National Council.

Sir Arthur Pearson was the first to endorse the CNIB at a high level by agreeing to become its first honorary president. His Excellency the Duke of Devonshire, Governor General of Canada at the time, became the CNIB's first patron, and with the exception of the years 1959 to 1976, every governor general since has accorded his or her patronage to the CNIB. Following suit, the lieutenant-governors of the provinces graciously serve as patrons of the geographic divisions.

Although the founders' reach was considerable and stretched well into the future, the CNIB was not the only rehabilitation agency for the blind in Canada. In 1936, when joint efforts to secure enabling legislation from the federal government were reaching their climax, there were no fewer than eighty-three representatives from associations "of" and "for" the blind as signatories. Some of these associations had existed well before 1918 and, in some cases, were well-established. The Montreal Association for the Blind and L'Institut Nazareth, both based in Quebec, were operating, as were the provincial schools in Ontario and Nova Scotia.

In several cities, such as Winnipeg, Ottawa, Toronto, and Halifax, industrial programs had been established to employ blind workers in the manufacture of brooms, brushes, mattresses, baskets, and leather goods.

Enterprising blind entrepreneurs had started piano tuning and shoe repair businesses. Poultry farming and later market gardening were also viable sources of employment.

For younger blind men and women who were graduating from schools for the blind, careers in music were becoming increasingly popular. However, blind people would remain barred from careers in the professions, such as law, medicine, politics, and teaching, for many years to come.

On the streets of large cities, however, there were no barriers to begging, and blind beggars were as common in Canada as in other cities around the world. The CNIB was facing a tradition dating as far back as the Quinze-Vingts ("fifteen score"), the first institution for the blind in the world. Founded by King Louis IX in thirteenth-century Paris as a hospice for three hundred knights blinded during the Crusades, the Quinze-Vingts remained a shelter and hospice for blind Parisians without family or property for centuries. Blind French beggars often enjoyed the patronage of the king and even wore specially designed robes to signal their privileged status.

The CNIB, however, was determined to move these men off the street and into gainful employment. The fact that begging could be more profitable than a low-paying job, however, was certainly a disincentive to the men. In September 1918, the CNIB National Council voted that no apprentices or workmen would be admitted to its workshops that were carrying on other lines of occupation of which the institute disapproved, or whose occupation was, in reality, mendicancy.

So this was the reality for blind people in Canada in the summer of 1918. For the CNIB, the focus was on Toronto, where the founders lived and the CNIB charter took root.

PEARSON HALL

At about the same time as the First World War was ending, in November 1918, Baker learned that the federal government held a significant special fund that had accrued from the surplus in the operation of the military canteen. The Governor General was charged with the discretionary responsibility of dispersing these funds. He selected provincial representation to assist in this task, and following a carefully crafted strategy, Baker and Wood obtained a $50,000

grant that represented 10 percent of the fund. They used $12,000 of the money to purchase a fine property in a fashionable neighborhood at 186 Beverley Street in downtown Toronto. Built in 1876

Public Testimonial

IN HONOR OF

Canadian Soldiers Blinded in the War

AND

Sir Arthur Pearson, Bart., G.B.E.
Founder of St. Dunstan's

UNDER THE AUSPICES OF

THE CANADIAN NATIONAL INSTITUTE FOR THE BLIND

MASSEY HALL
TUESDAY, JANUARY 7TH, 1919, AT 8 P.M.

Chairman
HON. W. J. HANNA, K.C.

Speakers
SIR ARTHUR PEARSON, BART., G.B.E.
HON. SIR WILLIAM HEARST, K.C.M.G.
HON. SIR JAMES LOUGHEED, K.C.M.G.
CAPTAIN E. A. BAKER, M.C., Croix de Guerre

Musical Programme
Mr. Colin O'More, Tenor   48th Highlanders' Band

Program cover for gala evening held at Massey Hall, January 1919.

by George Brown, a father of Canadian Confederation and founder of the *Globe* newspaper, the Second Empire mansion was refurbished as a rehabilitation centre modelled on St Dunstan's. Named Pearson Hall, in honour of Sir Arthur, the facility was opened in January 1919, with Sir Arthur himself in attendance.

The occasion was marked by a sold-out benefit gala, called a public testimonial, held at Massey Hall. The evening's entertainment included the singing of patriotic songs such as "The Maple Leaf Forever" and "Land of Hope and Glory" and addresses by special guest speakers including Prime Minister of Ontario Sir William Hearst, Minister of Soldiers' Civil Re-Establishment Sir James Lougheed, Edwin Baker, and Sir Arthur Pearson. The 48th Highlanders' Band performed.

Financial arrangements for the veterans who received training at Pearson Hall were as follows:

Each returned soldier on pay and allowance under the Department of Soldiers Civil Re-Establishment taking training at Pearson Hall, shall pay $25 a month during his residence at Pearson Hall, said amount to be held in trust and presented to him in a lump sum at the end of his period of training; soldiers who have graduated from St Dunstan's may enter Pearson Hall, free of charge for a period of one month, which period may be extended to three months at the discretion of the Institute authorities; for a longer period they shall pay $25 a month for board.

The seed money to develop the programs was drawn from the $50,000 grant, and the policy to establish a user fee was introduced as part of the training requirement.

Within a year or two, an annex was constructed, and Pearson Hall would house a library and teaching rooms, in addition to being the site of the CNIB's national headquarters. Because there was no room for a workshop for serious voca-

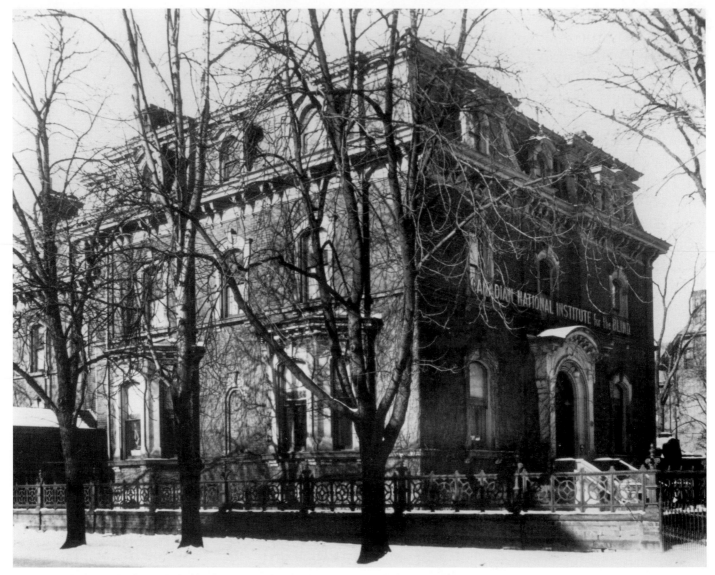

Pearson Hall, 186 Beverley Street, Toronto.

tional training, Holmes was authorized to find suitable space nearby, and in February 1919, a portion of the front end of the east side of premises at 455 King Street West was set aside for vocational training of the men.

Before this time, veterans had received some support from the Canadian Women's Association for

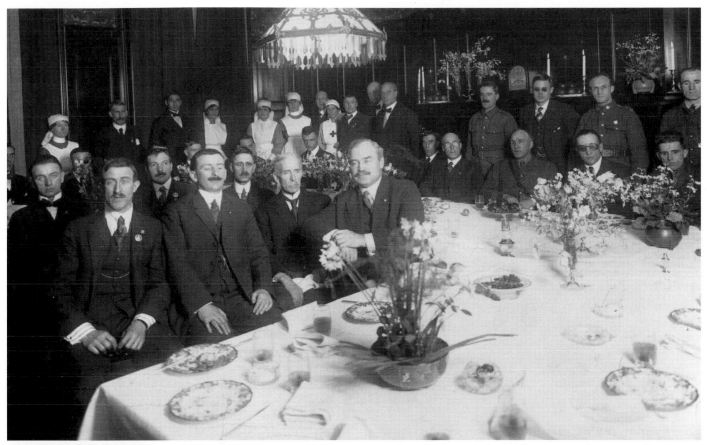

Banquet held at Pearson Hall to mark the official opening of the CNIB facility in 1919.

the Welfare of the Blind, which held tag days to raise money and organized dances, teas, and other social programs at the Christie Street Veterans' Hospital in Toronto. This association became the first auxiliary to the CNIB.

The impetus and ability to secure resources for blinded veterans accelerated the CNIB's growth.

In the early years, the war-blinded had access to more immediate and comprehensive programs than did civilians. This dual approach to service provision, although understandable, actually created two classes of clients within the CNIB and, ultimately, within Canadian society in general because those who had been blinded in war had access to special considerations such as pensions and allowances for personal care, travel, and technical devices like braille writing tools that civilians did not enjoy.

However, as services were developed and expanded and personnel were trained, most blind adults in Canada acquired access to services that were comparable to those the veterans were receiving.

Within one year of operation it was evident a decentralized management structure would be essential if a national organization were to be established and governed effectively. From the start, two unique approaches were adopted, and these are reflected in the institute's bylaws.

National Council created divisional boards of management with defined geographic areas to oversee CNIB operations. Local district advisory boards were then formed, extending the reach of the national organization further and deeper into the communities. The practice of a central authority, the national office, making policy decisions and providing operational direction remained constant.

On May 31, 1919, the young organization held its first annual general meeting, and the progress and achievements reported were nothing short of remarkable.

Speaking as president, Lew Wood thanked individuals for their contributions, named the key players in the CNIB's founding, and credited blind people with having been instrumental in the organization's work, including that done by the Free Library for the Blind. He also mentioned that the institute's membership stood at 734, which included 156 sighted people and 578 blind people, undoubtedly consumers or clients. (Over time, this balance in membership was reversed, and eventually blind people on the membership roll were the minority.) Approximately six thousand blind people were reported across Canada.

Other highlights of the report included the news that the CNIB's honorary president, Sir Arthur Pearson, had opened Pearson Hall, where twenty-five blinded veterans, graduates of St Dunstan's, had hosted a dinner in his honour. Sir Arthur had given public talks in Toronto, Hamilton, Ottawa, and Montreal and although the plan had been to invite him to return in

1920, he was unable to pay another visit.

The following programs were listed as having been up and running by May 31, 1919:

1. The number of men blinded in the First World War was reported as 125, 100 of whom returned to Canada, while the others remained in England. Captain Robert Thompson was appointed superintendent of the Blinded Soldiers Department, which later became known as the after-care program. The department was shown to have raised $4,852.66, recognizing the separate stream not only of services but also of financial reporting.

2. Registration of blind and visually impaired persons was detailed as to eye condition, disease, and pertinent personal information. The object was that "a register of the blind becomes a background and foundation not only for a study of their problems but for the practical handling thereof." Other applications cited included cause, hygienics, eugenics, safety, legislation, and study. (In the first year of the CNIB's operation, 1,521 blind Canadians, 926 male and 595 female, were registered with the organization. Three hundred and eighty-six were reported as active clients, not library patrons. By the year 2000, one hundred thousand people were registered as active clients. Although much of the same data have been collected over the years, little research has ever been undertaken. In respect to causes of blindness and disease, epidemiologists agree that the scientific basis for empirical research would be difficult, if not impossible, given the variance in reporting over the generations, and the evolution of medical knowledge.)

3. At the outset, fieldwork was described as "census work" and "social work." "Ambassadors," as the staff were described, spilled over into the range of services

from fundraising to rehabilitation in its various forms. The field worker became an "on-site agent," a model that is in place today, although the name is no longer in use.

4. Industrial departments for both men and women were established in Toronto. The men focused on manufacturing various products, and the women worked in craft and sewing trades. In the first year, there was only one women's workshop, with twenty-four people in the program. With sales of $997, the activity was rather limited. Knitted socks were sold by the Robert Simpson Co., and understandably, summer sales were reported to be slow. By contrast, the men's workshop had generated sales of $6,437. A much smaller program, boot repairs, operated at Pearson Hall by the veterans, had generated $13.15, not a high return.

5. The library had been very active, reporting that 744 items were circulated among 600 readers each month, the only cost to subscribers being that of the two-cent postage stamp on the letter requesting service. As the creation of braille music required paid transcribers, however, a modest fee, the second user fee, was passed on the blind musicians.

6. Of a salaried staff of twenty-seven at the National Office and Ontario Division, sixteen were home teachers. The role of the home teacher is so important it will be explored in more detail in a later chapter.

7. The Women's Auxiliary of the CNIB was replicated throughout the country. Women with social consciences, all well-established in their home communities, volunteered for a variety of tasks, ranging from fundraising to duties described as "social relief, prevention of blindness, support to the women's industrial department, entertainment and recreation." In a report,

Holmes described their work as "their labour of love."

8. Blindness prevention, one of the organization's founding objects, involved the medical community, so a nurse had been recruited in February 1919.

9. Fifty cases of sight-impaired children and adults were served.

The annual report also set out a detailed set of accounts audited by the Price Waterhouse firm of chartered accountants. H.D. Burns, honorary treasurer of the CNIB and chairman of the Bank of Nova Scotia, held the funds.

The balance sheet showed assets of $98,938, offset by liabilities in the same amount.

The operating budget for the first year totalled an impressive $118,000 with direct expenditures of $48,481. Revenue came from tag days that raised $41,000, donations of more than $50,000, and government grants of $10,000.

Interestingly, the names of all donors, regardless of the size of their donation, are listed in the annual report. Several personal and corporate gifts were sizeable, given the dollar values of the day, and others, while smaller, were nonetheless welcome and meaningful. Founding member Baker is shown to have donated $5, the Women's Christian Temperance Union of Toronto donated $3.50, and Claire Ghilcig, whoever she was, donated 50 cents.

The CNIB had organized a cooperative fundraising arrangement with Britain's National Institute for the Blind, later known as the Royal National Institute for the Blind (RNIB). Evelyn Cowan coordinated a joint appeal that raised $14,205 net. After the deduction of expenses, which were not specified, each organization received half, or $5,543. This arrangement with the RNIB remained in place for a few years.

By 1920, the CNIB had established operating divisions in Atlantic Canada, called the Maritime division, and Ontario. The western part of the country, thanks to the efforts of Holmes, now had a CNIB presence, too, with British Columbia and Alberta forming the Western division and

Saskatchewan and Manitoba making up the Central Western division. Although Newfoundland did not join the Dominion of Canada until 1949 it was served by the CNIB as the Newfoundland division at least by the 1930s.

With the formation of each division, a local board of management, elected from among leading volunteers, was put in place. These boards, although elected locally, were subject to the requirements and policies of National Council, and their membership was ratified annually by National Council.

This management structure, which allows for direct control from the institute's centre, remains in effect to this day and, with the possible exception of religious institutions, is unique in the Canadian not-for-profit sector.

A parallel structure exists at the organization's senior management level. In the beginning, the CNIB's top job was the director; in 1931, this was changed to managing director, a term still used in Britain today and one that reflected the British influence on the founders. (Titles, however, have been modernized in accordance with the times and North American naming conventions. The managing director's title was changed to president and CEO, and the president of National Council then became known as its chair. In 1997, National Council was restructured and renamed the Board of Directors.) The managing director appointed or "posted" a superintendent (now called the executive director) in each division. The reporting structure was clearly on a solid line, including compensation and term of employment.

To a degree, this model reflected a military style of governance and administration, and as recently as the 1980s an organizational chart was referred to as the "chain of command." Over time, the provincial boards assumed greater control over their affairs, including a role in the recruitment of their own executive directors.

With the exception of New Zealand, no other Commonwealth country of the day adopted this organizational structure, with the result that in many countries, blindness service organizations became competitive duplications of one another.

In Canada (although not in Quebec, where the situation was quite different), the CNIB was the sole organization offering a broad spectrum of rehabilitation services for the blind.

THE ONTARIO DIVISION

In June 1919, given the diversity of service and the residential and workshop operations, the leadership in Toronto decided to establish the province of Ontario as a division separate from the national office. The work of Pearson Hall and the library, however, were not to be included in the new division. Guy Robertson was appointed the first superintendent of the Ontario division, on trial for six months, at a salary of $1,500 per year. Robertson resigned in December of that year and was replaced in February 1920 by M.I. Tynam, who was appointed acting superintendent on the recommendation of the Ontario Board of Management. The word *acting* was removed from his title in May.

By September, however, the Ontario division seems to have been in trouble, and National Council resolved that the offices of the division be removed from 142 College Street to the head office at 36 King Street East, that effective September 15, 1920, the Ontario division be abolished, that the work of the home teachers and field workers being supervised by Tynam be assumed by the director, and that the supervision of the business be undertaken directly by the national business manager. This rather dramatic reversal came about because it was felt that the business affairs of the division needed to be more centralized.

The result of this reversal was, in effect, to make Baker managing director of both the national and Ontario operations. For thirty years, until the re-establishment of the Ontario division in 1952, the national office exercised direct control over the division and had access to Ontario's sizeable sector of Canada's wealth, population, and CNIB client base.

This certainly strengthened the notion that what was good for Ontario would be good for the remainder of the national organization and vice versa.

Early on, the CNIB leadership made crucial decisions that would set the agenda for years to come. For example, from its inception, the CNIB has viewed the prevention of blindness as a vital part of its mandate and has always played a role in creating awareness of vision health on the national and international stages; policies, advocacies, organizational growth, and program development entrenched within the first five years of the organization's founding have continued, in many cases, to the present day.

Writing in the CNIB's first annual report of 1919, Holmes laid a foundation of the importance of blindness prevention as one of the institute's cornerstone programs:

> There is nothing so important in the scheme of things, and nothing that appeals so strongly to the interest, sympathy and judgment of workers in the cause of the blind as the prevention of blindness itself.
>
> We are not only anxious to be of the greatest and most practical service to those who have been unfortunate enough to lose their sight, but we are just as anxious to minimize to the lowest possible point, the number of those who, in future, shall meet with a similar loss.

Holmes might well have ended his observation at this point, but he had further thoughts on the matter: "Not only is this human and Christian, but it is economic as well. The cost to the community of the education of a blind child is many fold that of the education of the sighted child."

This view echoed what Egerton Ryerson, the educator, had reported to the Ontario Legislature half a century earlier. Holmes went on: "The loss to the community in the limited efficiency of the average blind workman as compared to the average sighted workman is tremendous. And all this with regard to the deprivation to the individual himself."

As part of the CNIB's early operations, registering blind people provided an immediate and accurate database that proved extremely useful in applying for government grants, developing and delivering programs, and enabling greater access to medical care when remedial assistance was required. At the same time, the registration process gave the institute proprietary knowledge of its clients.

The CNIB also negotiated an agreement with the Dominion Bureau of Statistics that every ten years, the census takers would be paid a per capita bonus for identifying and reporting blind people who might benefit from receiving CNIB services. (The census takers were paid 2.5 cents per sighted person, but 10 cents if the person was blind.) This practice continued until 1951, by which time the CNIB had its own resources in place to identify potential clients. However, this was an effective and early method in public administration to identify and classify a specific disability group.

Although war-blinded veterans, and the facility established for them, marked the earliest days of the CNIB, the organization also endeavoured to serve civilian men and women. By November 1918, premises at 42 Adelaide Street West had been rented for the Industrial School for Blind Women,

and separate residences for men and women were soon acquired, establishing the CNIB as a provider of residential care.

Workshop programs administered by the organization provided employment for blind people, but labour relations were not always harmonious, as this excerpt from a letter, dated July 15, 1920, from Director Holmes to A.A. Archibald, broom shop manager in Vancouver, shows. The letter, which reveals something of the CNIB's growing pains, had been written in response to a complaint after the national office took a unilateral decision to close the shop:

I may say that the demand of the men in your Shop of some few weeks ago for an increase of remuneration naming fifteen dollars a week as a vocational allowance, and the attitude of Carlson in particular, demanding a dollar a dozen for winding brooms and declaring that whether he could or not would not attempt to turn out more than three dozen a day, etc. have all been elements rather contributing towards a feeling of, I might almost say, disgust with the ingratitude and lack of appreciation of the whole situation on the part of those who would take such a position as above mentioned. Furthermore, there has been trouble in other places, and to make a long story short, the Committee is getting pretty well fed up with the Bolshevism of those who, instead of being grateful for the benefits which have been made available for them are disposed to make more and more unpleasant-ness for all concerned the more benefits they derive.

It has been felt that some of them needed a lesson, that some of them had better be shown where they get off, that some of them had better be given an opportunity of consider-ing whether or not they are better off than they were before they came to us and than they will be when they leave us, and in other words, that the closing of one shop with the intimation that others might follow would have a salutary effect upon all.

In other areas, however, the CNIB was making good progress. The CNIB and the Canadian National Library for the Blind amalgamated in December 1919, and a home teaching program, to provide vocational instruction to adults, had been set up by January of 1920.

Employment and vocational programs were becoming more for-malized as Joseph Clunk, of Youngstown, Ohio, was engaged in December 1927 as placement offi-cer on a one-month trial basis. By February of the following year, in view of Clunk's success in placing blind individuals in industry, it was recommended that he should be engaged as placement officer on the regular staff of the institute.

Catering and "dry stand" or canteen operations became a source of sustained employment for blind individuals, and by the 1940s they had expanded into a very large commercial operation for the CNIB.

THE FOUNDERS IN LATER YEARS

The CNIB's founders, meanwhile, who had accomplished so much in a relatively short period of time, went on with their lives.

George Plaxton, the lawyer who had drafted the CNIB's articles of incorporation and presented the letter from the undersecretary of state at the first meeting of National Council, returned to his law practice. Some years later, he was elected to National Council, and as he approached the end of his life he made a $1,000 contribution to the Bayview Avenue building campaign in 1954. He died in 1955.

The steadfast Alexander Viets, who had been Baker's roommate at St Dunstan's, served on the Blinded Soldiers Welfare Committee and remained a friend and confidant of Baker until Viets' death in 1949.

Sherman Swift, who assumed the role of head of the library and publishing department when the Canadian National Library for the Blind amalgamated with the CNIB in 1919, held that position until his death on May 27, 1947.

He gained international stature as an academic, linguist, and authority on braille codes and publication. He also oversaw the introduction of the "talking book" in the 1930s. A handwritten letter to him from Canadian humorist Stephen Leacock granting permission — "that goes without saying" — to have *Sunshine Sketches of a Little Town* brailled reflects the scope of his contacts. He was awarded an honorary doctorate from his alma mater, McGill University, in 1936.

Charles Carruthers, the blind lawyer and osteopath, was hired in 1918 to teach braille at Pearson Hall at the rate of $2.50 per day, three hours per day. By September, he was being paid $1,000 per year for full-time braille instruction. He was a member of the first National Council, and in 1950 he was re-elected to the council after some years' absence. He was named honorary president in 1973. The last surviv-

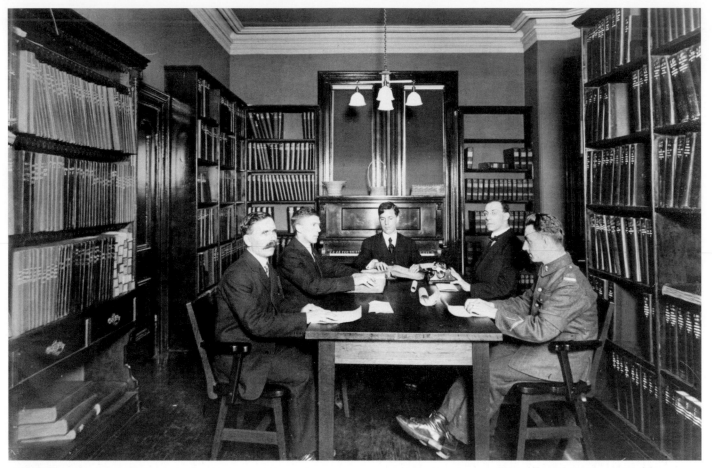

CNIB founding member Charles Carruthers teaches braille in the reading room.

ing founder, he lived for a time in the CNIB's Clarkewood Residence and died at the age of ninety on May 14, 1976.

Dr. Charles Dickson experienced a somewhat difficult association with the CNIB. At the very first meeting of the institute, on March 18, 1918, he was elected president and appointed general secretary at a salary of $1,200 per year. On August 6, 1918, just six months after his election as the organization's first president, he submitted a letter of resignation to National Council, paving the way for fellow founder Lew Wood to be elected to that office. Dr. Dickson's

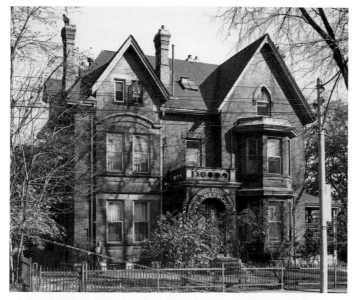

The Clarkewood Women's Residence at 331 Sherbourne Street in Toronto was open from July 1920 to February 1956.

letter, it should be noted, does not indicate any malice or regret and is generous and eloquent, as this excerpt shows:

> When you did me the exceptional honour of electing me to be both President and General Secretary of the Institute, I accepted with the distinct understanding that when organization was complete, and someone more widely known than myself was available for the office of President, I should be permitted to resign the office and devote my entire energies and time to the duties of your General Secretary.
>
> I feel that the time is now opportune, and the ideal man available for the desired change. I also feel sure that you will agree with me.
>
> I therefore take pleasure in formally tendering my resignation as President and asking the privilege of nominating as my successor, Mr. L.M. Wood, who needs no words of commendation.
>
> I bespeak for my successor that loyalty, enthusiasm, and hearty co-operation, which you have ever accorded myself, and which I have appreciated more deeply than I can express.

In December 1918, Dickson was appointed chairman of the Blinded Soldier's Committee, but by May of 1919, his failing health was attributed to "his devotion to the interests of the Institute since its creation"; he was given a three-month leave of absence, and at the end of that period was superannuated at an annuity of $750.

Perhaps Dickson's combative nature exhausted his constructive involvement with the leadership of the institute. He may also have fallen on hard financial times as his health declined. Much older than his colleagues, he died on July 9, 1938, in Toronto. Many years later, an invoice for his funeral, presumably paid for the management of the day, was discovered in the CNIB archives.

Sir Arthur Pearson, who had been so influential to several of the founders through his work with St Dunstan's, died in London in 1921 at the age of fifty-six. His widow, Lady Pearson, later consented to the use of his name for the Sir Arthur Pearson Association of War Blinded (SAPA), an exclusive group whose membership is limited to those who were blinded in war. (A separate history of Canada's war-blinded soldiers and their proprietary association is being written for publication in 2005.)

Lewis M. Wood, CBE, who took over from Dickson as the second president of the CNIB in August 1918, served in that role with great distinction for thirty-four years. In reply to a letter of condolence after Wood's death in 1954, Baker described him as "a tower of strength and sagacity through the years."

In August 1918, Baker was asked to head a newly established department for the training and after-care of Canada's war veterans, which had been set up by the federal government; while doing this job he also remained active with the CNIB as a vice-president. By 1920, it was evident that his energy, talent, and leadership skills were desperately needed at the CNIB, and in October he took up his new position as general secretary. His starting salary is discreetly left blank in the National Council minutes.

Baker, who had been a serving lieutenant when he was injured and returned to Canada, had been gazetted a captain in 1917. In

1938 he was offered the honorary rank of lieutenant-colonel, after which he was usually called Colonel Baker. He spent the rest of his career with the CNIB and received worldwide accolades in recognition of his work. He retired in 1962 to Parrott's Bay near Kingston, Ontario, just a few miles from his birthplace, where he died suddenly on April 7, 1968.

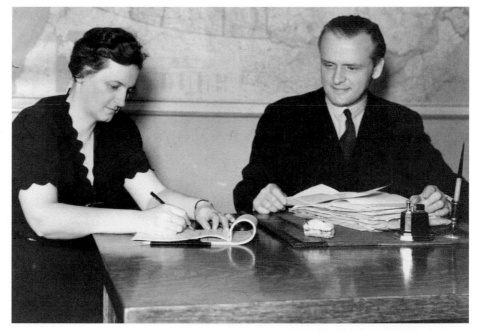

Grace Worts was Edwin Baker's loyal secretary for decades. They are shown here in 1923.

Charles Holmes served out his five-year contract from 1918 to 1923 and then some. However, early on it became evident that his enthusiasm to fulfill his aggressive mandate would put him on a direct collision course with council members and the scarce resources available to them.

Holmes had been directed to move quickly to develop both industrial training and rehabilitation programs and had been reassured, in writing, that the financial resources he would need to carry out this work would be made available. Apparently, this did not happen. In a long and detailed letter to National Council, Holmes took great exception on two issues. First, he complained bitterly that some unnamed person had countermanded his decisions, thereby undermining his authority and credibility. He also complained that sizeable capital purchases for the workshops had been placed, some in the United States, and then summarily cancelled. Holmes then reminded his employers that they had committed to secure the resources. The response to his letter, if there was one, is not known, but the tone and content of Holmes's letter would not have sat well with the senior volunteer leadership.

The July 15, 1920, letter written by Holmes to A.A. Archibald in Vancouver discussing the details of the closure of the broom shop hints at further growing differences in strategy and management style, particularly between Holmes and Wood, the president of National Council. Holmes implies that Wood's sending a telegram on July 12 advising that the workshop was to be closed immediately had been precipitous and insensitive to the employees: "I do not feel that the summary closing without consultation and notice of so important an undertaking as the Vancouver broom shop was well advised, and I have had no hesitation in so stating."

With an understanding of the implications of the closing from a public relations point of view that was well ahead of his time, Holmes muses further that the news might occasion a negative public reaction that could be harmful to the young organization's image.

Referring to the touse [sic] which the men will no doubt raise over their dismissal, Mr. Wood has taken the position that it will really be to the interest of the cause in the long run that they should do as much rowing as they are disposed and even that they should go to members of the British Columbia legislature if they like … he feels that the publicity and agitation created by this situation will occasion a greater readiness on the part of the public and perhaps particularly the legislature to consider adequate local financial support … I have pointed out … it may result in quite a contrary point of view on the part of the local people.

Holmes clearly thought Wood was mistaken if he thought that by encouraging the blind workers to go public with their complaints the government of British Columbia would respond by increasing fund-

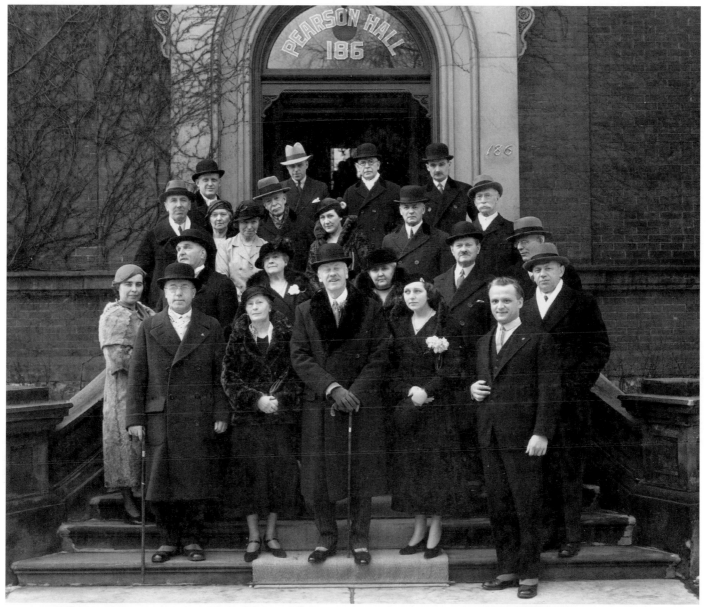

In 1933, Governor General Sir Vere Brabazon Ponsonby, ninth Earl of Bessborough, front row centre, visited Pearson Hall. Edwin Baker is on the far right, front row, and Alexander Viets is on the far left, front row. Standing between the governor general and Baker is Lady Virginia Kemp.

ing to the CNIB. Earlier in the letter Holmes noted that the British Columbia government had introduced in its budget an item of $40,000 for the education of blind pupils, with minimum funding for other programs. If Wood, likely supported by others on the council, thought his strategy would work, he was mistaken. For the next eighty years, compared to other provinces, successive British Columbia governments provided only minimal grants to the CNIB. Holmes appears to have been right.

As his term of employment drew to a close in June 1923, National Council "resolved that the appreciation of the Council be extended to Mr. Holmes for his splendid services in laying a foundation for work for the blind in Canada and regrets that he is severing his connection with the Institute and further that a bonus of $500 be handed him with the best wishes of the Council for his future success."

But his relationship with the CNIB was not over yet. In September he was appointed in an advisory capacity in connection with prevention of blindness in Canada, at a salary of $125 per month, with engagement terminable by either party on three months' notice. Unfortunately, the arrangement did not last long, and by January National Council had decided to give Holmes his three months' notice.

When Holmes left the organization to return to his home in the United States, Sherman Swift was charged with organizing a tribute to him. The National Archives in Ottawa holds a detailed account of the gratitude many blind people felt toward him.

On May 3, 1940 Baker wrote a touching tribute to Holmes, who had recently died, praising his work in the development of the home teaching movement in Canada: "While adults in Canada may continue through accident or illness to lose their sight, and while the home teaching services of the Institute are maintained for service to them, the foresight and wisdom of the late Charles W. Holmes will ever be gratefully remembered."

By 1926, the Canadian Federation of the Blind, with Philip Layton of the MAB as its president, would begin to galvanize significant and effective opposition to the CNIB, which would go on for the next thirty years. This opposition included mounting formal protests to governments on credibility issues, fundraising, and sphere of authority. This was, in many respects, an expression of the fact that a national organization was simply not welcome in a provincial jurisdiction.

Because four of the founders, Baker, Wood, Swift, and Carruthers, would remain involved with the CNIB for many decades, the organization stayed with the vision and drive that had launched it. Determination and leadership were there in abundance.

Resistance to the CNIB, however, was real, resources were scarce, and public policy was slow to change. Negative public attitudes toward blindness were deeply entrenched.

The CNIB's early successes remain true victories in Canadian philanthropy. But did the strength and vision of its founders also sow the seeds of paternalism and a monopolistic style of ownership?

Some would say, yes, they did.

CHAPTER 4
That All May Read

"For the library to have to close would be a terrible blow to the Blind, especially to me," wrote Kitty Curry in November 1914. "I don't know what I would do if it were not for our library. I am of a melancholy disposition, and as I must depend solely on myself for reading, if I am deprived of what literature we have in raised print, I fear to think what would become of me."

From ancient script carved in stone to the invention of braille in the nineteenth century to the interactive computer screens of the millennium, access to information across the centuries for people who are blind, visually impaired, or deaf-blind has been both a challenge and a source of joy and opportunity.

It is through touch and sound that literacy comes to life. Blind poets in ancient days recited or sang their creative work from memory. Blind people are relative newcomers to the world of literacy; in contrast to the sighted world, blind people have been able to access and retrieve information for fewer than two centuries, starting with the invention and refinement of the braille system by Louis Braille in about 1830 in France. Knowledge through recorded sound followed about fifty years later, beginning in the 1880s with the invention of the phonograph, and now includes audio tape, compact discs, and computer systems.

Braille into the Next Millennium is an excellent resource on the history and applications of braille. In his foreword to the book, Frank Kurt Cylke, director of the National Library Service for the Blind and Physically Handicapped (NLS), a division of the U.S. Library of Congress, writes: "With a tactile medium such as braille comes literacy — spelling, writing, and broad communication possibilities are open and available. With literacy comes the possibility of freedom. With freedom comes the possibility of endless achievement — from pleasant living to significant social contributions ..."

Some people have suggested that Information Age technology will make braille obsolete. The reality, however, is that for people who are blind or visually impaired, braille and digital audio technology can and should work together as the means to accessible information.

In Canada, the idea to teach braille and distribute brailled books in both French and English was imported from Europe and the United States by schools for the blind as early as 1870, and by the late nineteenth century some braille books were being circulated by the schools' libraries to adult readers. There were very few patrons, however, because very few people could actually read braille. An adult blind person who had not been fortunate enough to have attended a school for the blind, or who became blind as an adult, would not have had access to instruction in braille until the first decade of the twentieth century, as specific organizations with personnel qualified to teach braille emerged.

Founded at a meeting of blind men and women in Toronto on November 9, 1906, the Canadian Free Library for the Blind (CFLB) was the third institution in Canada to offer a circulating library specifically for the blind, writes Janet B. Friskey in *History of the Book in Canada*, a three-volume, interdisciplinary work with many authors.

The CFLB was the long-held dream of Edgar Bertram Freel Robinson, who had begun lending copies of his own braille books out of his home in Markham, Ontario. Robinson died suddenly in 1908 of typhoid, and his sighted wife, Marion, took over as librarian. The CFLB, which had changed its name in 1916 to the Canadian National Library for the Blind, merged in 1919 with the newly formed Canadian National Institute for the Blind.

In 1874, twenty-two nations were signatories to an international treaty allowing for matter for the blind to be delivered at no charge to blind people. By the year 2000, 180 countries, almost every country in the world, had become part of this agreement under the auspices of the Universal Postal Union.

In 1898, the Canadian Parliament amended the Post Office Act to permit the delivery of braille materials through the post at no cost to a blind individual or an institution serving blind people. Canada takes credit for being the first country to enact such legislation.

Under current Canada Post regulations, literature for the blind is available free of charge to blind people and recognized institutions for the blind. Only the following items can be mailed as literature for the blind: items impressed in braille or similar raised type; plates for printing literature for the blind; tapes and records posted by the blind; and recording tapes, records, and special writing paper intended solely for the use of the blind when mailed by, or addressed to, a recognized institution for the blind.

However, trends within some countries toward privatization, such as the use of courier services to collect and deliver mail and parcels, could pose a serious threat to this entitlement over the long term.

By 1920, the CNIB library was producing and distributing an ever-increasing number of braille volumes and materials in English. L'Institut Nazareth in Montreal was also developing materials in French. These libraries operated independently and relied on donations from the private sector. Only the schools for the blind had access to public funding from the education budgets of the provinces where the schools were located —

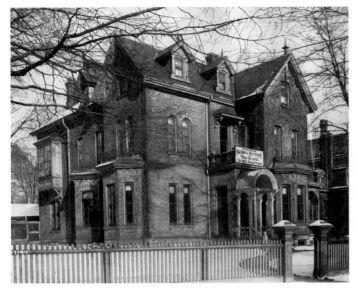

The CNIB's library department was located at 142 College Street in Toronto.

Nova Scotia, Ontario, and later British Columbia.

In the British North America Act of 1867, culture — and its expression through libraries — is clearly set out as a provincial responsibility. Within the provinces, local or municipal governments operate branch libraries funded through local property taxes, provincial granting mechanisms, or a combination of funding approaches. Virtually nowhere, at any level of government, has financial support as a fundamental principle or legislated entitlement existed to fund private libraries for the blind, wherever they may be located. Sporadic provincial funding for the production and distribution of alternate format materials, like braille or audio tape, began in the late 1970s in response to growing pressure for accessible information, led by the CNIB. These funds, allocated grudgingly, were used mainly to create educational materials, with some leisure reading thrown in.

A hit-or-miss system of providing grants and the purchase of service arrangements have led to a fragmented library picture for blind people in every part of Canada. By the 1970s, public libraries began to take notice, and modest collections of large print and audio books were made available. Public libraries, however, do not lend braille books or magazines. Provincial departments of education and some universities do provide educational material in an accessible format. Unfortunately, jurisdictional issues among provinces militate against a national coordinated approach.

The true conundrum, discriminatory in nature, is that a tax-supported public library service is

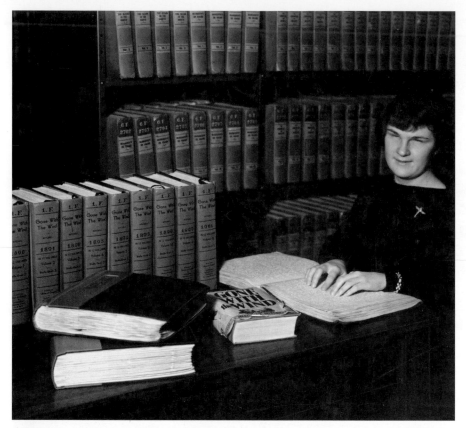

Mary Edwards sets out to read all twelve volumes of *Gone With the Wind* in braille.

The National Library of Canada, located in Ottawa and established by Parliament in 1953, is a federal cultural agency responsible for collecting and preserving Canada's published heritage. Put another way, the library's major role is to acquire, preserve, and promote Canadiana, which is part of the published and oral heritage of this country.

From 1960 onwards, the National Library of Canada has struggled to support and encourage development of adequate and accessible library services for the blind and millions of other Canadians unable to read print.

available to the citizens of the nation, generally free of charge — but blind people, taxed at the same rate as their sighted neighbours, do not receive the same benefits. Taxation of the blind and the continuing barriers to equitable accessibility border on a national shame and are analogous to the concept of taxation without representation.

Fuzzy mandates and the lack of political will on the part of the federal government have ensured the statutory ineligibility for private libraries for the blind to receive public funding.

Despite these nearly insurmountable obstacles, the CNIB has grown and has achieved the status of a world-class private service organization. The multi-million-dollar budget required to serve the one hundred thousand CNIB clients who are entitled to receive library service and the 3 million Canadians who have difficulty reading print is an annual exercise in financial survival. Hundreds of qualified, committed volunteers work with highly specialized CNIB staff to produce braille books and music and to narrate or read audio materials. These dedicated individuals form the nucleus of the library program and are in large part responsible for its success.

The experiences among other developed nations vary, as do the standards of library services in the blindness field. Let's look at how the Americans do it.

In 1931, at the urging of Robert Irwin of the American Foundation for the Blind (AFB), U.S. President Herbert Hoover signed into law the Pratt-Smoot Act, which established a national free library service for blind people and called for $100,000 to be administered by the Library of Congress to provide blind adults with books. The AFB joined with the American Printing House for the Blind (APH) in Louisville,

Kentucky, and the Braille Institute in Los Angeles, California, to urge Congress to centralize the production and distribution of library services for the blind. This approach was viewed as cost-effective and efficient. In 1932, the first grant was voted from the treasury, and funding books for the blind continues to be part of the U.S. Library of Congress's annual budgeting process. In 1933

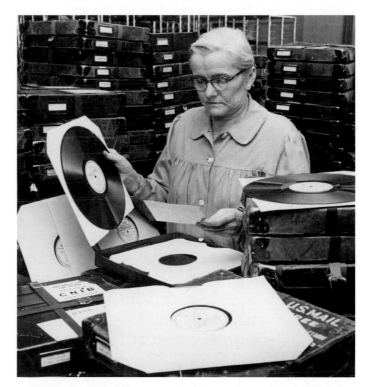

Mabel Eaglestone sorts long-play records in the CNIB's circulation department, 1961.

the act was amended to include talking books.

While private organizations produce supplementary materials, as do commercial sources, the National Library Service of the Library of Congress provides a leisure library for blind people unequalled anywhere in the world. Each year the NLS spends many millions of dollars on training braillists, producing braille books, periodicals, and music materials, and purchasing materials in all languages from many countries around the world. In 2003, with a budget of $50 million, the NLS produced 627 braille books, 2,059 audio books, 33 magazines in braille (408,000 copies), and recorded 45 magazine titles (4 million copies). Altogether, it shipped almost 2 million items to blind and visually impaired readers. The library runs fifty-seven regional libraries, seventy-seven sub-regional libraries, and two multi-state centres. It has 110 people on staff and has 38,000 braille and 728,000 audio readers registered. Its total collection is estimated at more than 23 million books and magazines in all formats.

In Canada, meanwhile, blind readers in every city and hamlet of the country have always relied on the postal service to deliver braille and audio books to their homes. In more remote areas, such as the far north, where air transport, replacing dog sleds, was required to deliver mail, the CNIB lobbied the post office to carry braille and audio books on the planes. This was eventually agreed to in the mid-1930s even though these bulky, heavy books took up precious space on the small aircraft of the day.

Delivering books to blind people in Newfoundland and Labrador posed a special challenge in the early days because although geographically part of the Canadian mainland, it was a British colony, and thus outside the jurisdiction of the Canadian postal service.

To describe a library for the blind as only a library is something of a misnomer and understates the scope of its operations beyond the lending of materials. The CNIB library in Toronto and similar libraries in Quebec are also manufacturing, storage, distribution, and retrieval centres. The operations are labour-intensive, time-consuming, and costly in both materials and plant facilities. Special training is required to produce these materials; costly equipment is needed for the production process. The Information Age, with its expectations of instant communication, and digital technologies have added to the complexity of the demands.

Although the computer revolution of the 1970s brought about the most radical change in the way braille is produced, stored, and distributed since it was invented in 1829, producing braille on paper, in the old-fashioned way, remains essential because electronic braille is limited to one word or one line at a time based on refreshable embossed pins that pop up and down. Until a breakthrough is found, electronic braille remains prohibitively expensive and unavailable to the majority of blind users.

TALKING BOOKS

Audio or talking books first appeared in North America in the early 1930s. Much earlier, in 1877, American inventor Thomas Edison filed a patent application for what came to be his favourite invention, the phonograph. In listing ten suggested applications for the new gadget, the far-seeing Edison stated, "the phonograph book which will speak to blind people without effort on their part." This application was listed second, ahead of music, which was fourth.

Sherman Swift, who was appointed secretary of the Free Library for the Blind on the death of Edgar Robinson and who went on to serve with distinction for many years as the CNIB librarian, ensured that blind Canadians would share in this revolutionary technology. Until then, one person, usually sighted, reading aloud to a blind person was the sole alternative to braille.

The AFB and the APH produced the first talking books in the United States, but some recorded books were also obtained by the CNIB from England. The books were recorded on heavy discs such as 78-rpm records and, later, LP (33 1/3) discs. These records, however, were specially adapted to be played at slower speeds than commercial applications so more material could be recorded on each disc. Special playback equipment was produced, and then discs and equipment were shipped to library users.

The discs were fragile and often arrived broken or damaged. Many did not survive delivery or the cold Canadian winters. In the early days of audio books, novels and magazines were recorded, but the quality of the recordings was very poor indeed. Gradually, educational and employment-related materials were included in the collections. As technology improved, accelerated by commercial broadcasting applications, the materials for the blind improved, including the capacity for local or individual production with the advent of the reel-to-reel tape recorder — never mind that it was bulky and heavy. By the 1950s, following engineering ingenuity from the Second World War, blind people who had the financial means had access to an ever expanding source of improved recording and playback equipment and consequently of audio materials.

The CNIB library moved from the large discs to a British six-track format known as the Clarke and Smith system. This system involved a large, sealed container that fit over an equally large and heavy playback machine. While this system could contain several books, it presented serious shipping and maintenance problems. The "tapette" was much smaller, as was the playback device, and contained a magnetic tape with eight tracks on which an entire book could be recorded.

The Clarke and Smith system was used in Canada for only about ten years until 1978. By then, the American NLS had developed a special system utilizing the standard cassette. The cassette was recorded on four tracks as opposed to the two tracks used commercially, and was replayed at half the normal playing speed.

Importantly, this meant that one hour of commercial recording time could be increased to six hours on the same cassette. The playback machine used in this system was designed and manufactured in the United States. Several countries, including Canada, Australia, and New Zealand, adopted this system, and books could be purchased or loaned between countries that shared the system and sought English titles.

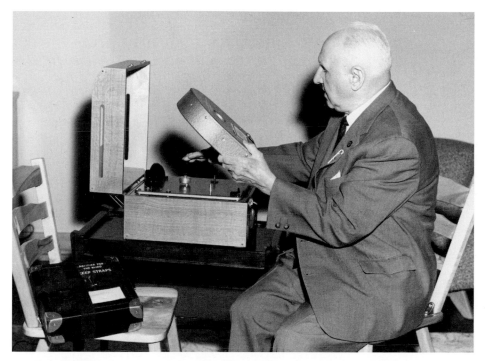

E.P. Hill, a guest at Fundy Hall Residence for the Blind in New Brunswick, uses a talking book machine, 1966.

The quality of the recorded books improved as recording equipment become more advanced, and production standards were developed that ensured a more enjoyable and realistic experience for the listener.

In other countries, the technologies and sound recording systems among libraries for the blind varied greatly. No international standard existed, and in developing countries, audio books were non-existent.

Affordability remains the critical issue, and the availability of power sources cannot be taken for granted. Braille remains the main alternative for the majority of the world's 180 million blind people.

In all these developments, the matter of copyright laws and ownership was taken into account. In Canada, copyright permission was obtained prior to producing any work either in braille or audio format. Other countries were also required to follow this practice. Exemption from this requirement took place in 1977 in Japan when legislation was enacted allowing for production of these materials. The U.S. Congress has since passed a similar law.

The CNIB played a leading role in obtaining amendments to the Copyright Act so that the making of braille, audio, and e-text copies

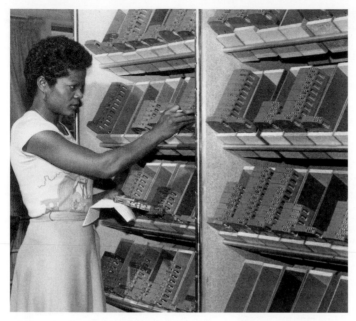

Shelving tapettes in the CNIB library, 1975.

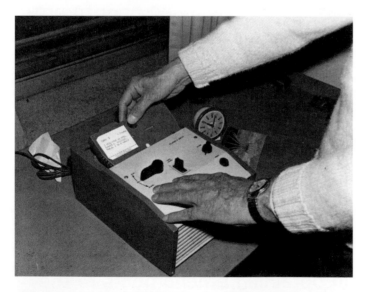

Clarke and Smith talking book machine.

of a work would not infringe on copyright. The amendment, passed in 1996, has sped up the process of providing copies in alternate formats since the library no longer has to wait for copyright permission.

AMATEUR RADIO CLUB

In the days before the Internet, there was amateur radio, or, as it was called, ham radio. In a 1978 interview with Paul O'Neill, national director of public relations, David Lloyd (VE3AW, or, as he preferred to refer to himself, VE3 — Awful Whisky), chair of the CNIB Amateur Radio Club for ten years, recounted the full history of the ham radio program in Canada and within the CNIB.

In that year, Lloyd said, there were more than a million hams around the world, and eighteen thousand in Canada. The number of blind hams has reached as many as six hundred.

From a small beginning in 1967, when sixteen Radio Society of Ontario members began sponsoring blind radio hams, interest in the hobby grew. By 1974, 363

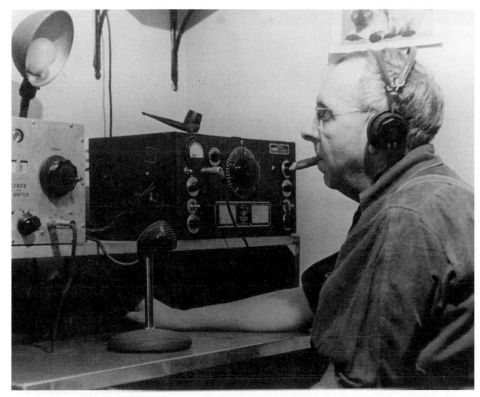

Hugh McCrea of Bathurst, New Brunswick, the first ham radio operator in the Maritime division, 1954.

safe, simple rigs that could be adjusted by touch and sound. The equipment was loaned to or purchased by the individual operator. To make the program affordable, equipment could be bought on a time plan at low rates. James Swail, a blind researcher with the National Research Council of Canada, designed special adaptations for the equipment so a blind ham could transmit and receive independently.

The work of the Radio Society of Ontario sponsors, and others, meant that blind people could communicate with thousands of radio hams across Canada and around the world. A ham shack was set up at BakerWood in Toronto, with the call letters VE3NIB.

sponsors across Canada were providing instruction, assembling hardware, installing equipment, and serving on technical committees. That year, there were 246 blind radio operators, 25 of whom were women, in Canada.

It was estimated that the sponsors put in thirty-six thousand hours on assembly alone to provide blind radio operators with

Over the years, blind radio operators were credited with assisting authorities and even saving lives in such emergency situations as floods, missing children, snow slides, heart attacks, and boating mishaps; many of these blind hams were honoured for their outstanding efforts.

Relatively small in number compared to other programs, the Amateur Radio Club has a loyal, dedicated following who spend countless hours enjoying pleasant conversations with "unseen" friends in every corner of the globe.

VOICEPRINT

Every morning, millions of people take a few moments to catch up on the world's affairs over the day's first cup of coffee. And they don't think much about it. For a blind person, however, this small ritual isn't so easy or enjoyable. Even if a sighted person is willing to read the paper to him, what he hears generally depends on what the reader thinks he would like to hear.

To solve this problem, forty years ago the Radio Reading Service (RRS) began in the United States when volunteers began reading newspapers and magazines for broadcast to blind subscribers. For copyright and other reasons, this transmission was received by a special receiver, and its range was limited. However, for the first time blind people could "read" print editions of newspapers. The material read was of necessity selective, and time schedules slotted in what would be read, on what day, and at what time of the day.

In 1970, the CNIB sent two staff members to study the program with a view to implementing a similar one in Canada. The result was that a small RRS was launched in Oakville, Ontario. However, there were few subscribers due to the cost of the receiver and the limited range of transmission, which could not fully cover the urban area of Toronto and surrounding cities.

In Quebec, a French-language reading service on cable was launched by La Magnétothèque, a private audio transcription service funded by the Quebec government.

In 1985, James Sanders, executive director of the CNIB's B.C.-Yukon division, was asked to chair a task force to study and make recommendations on how newspapers and magazines could be made accessible, in a timely manner, to blind people.

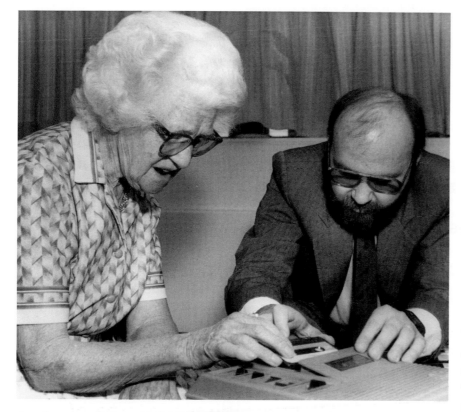

Robert Ganong, intake counsellor in the Nova Scotia–Prince Edward Island division, demonstrates a talking book machine to Susie Keen.

The far-reaching "Right to Know" report, released in 1988, led to the establishment in 1989 of the National Broadcast Reading Service (NBRS), a not-for-profit registered charity, to set up and operate VoicePrint, Canada's national reading service, which has been broadcasting twenty-four hours a day since December 1, 1990. Although the NBRS began as a CNIB initiative, and the key players in establishing it were CNIB volunteers Frances Cutler, Gerry Dirks, and Dayton Forman, it was intentionally created as an independent organization and was founded with a government grant of $500,000 over five years.

Licensed by the Canadian Radio-television and Telecommunications Commission (CRTC), VoicePrint depends upon hundreds of volunteers to produce full-text readings of published news stories for broadcast across Canada. The service reaches more than 8 million homes, and listeners can access VoicePrint via satellite, cable, and direct-to-home services, including the Internet at ~~voiceprint.ca~~ *AMI.CA* *

Most of each program day consists of verbatim readings of newspaper and magazine articles packaged into topical program segments. Business, sports,

~~Accessible~~ Media INC
AMI-Audio AMI-TV

health and science, lifestyles and leisure, regional news, and old-time radio shows are some of the other topics included in the program lineup. Programming in the national service is recorded at Toronto, Ottawa, Winnipeg, Calgary, Vancouver, and Victoria.

While VoicePrint's core target audience is blind or vision-impaired Canadians, more than five hundred thousand Canadians from all walks of life cite VoicePrint as their main source of news and information.

Throughout the 1990s the organization struggled financially, but under the dogged determination of its executive director, Bob Trimby, the CRTC agreed to impose an assessment on cable operators, which would provide a small funding base for VoicePrint.

To further support its mandate — to enhance access to visual media for vision- and print-restricted Canadians — in 1995 the NBRS launched its second division, AudioVision Canada (AVC), as an audio description production centre. Movies and TV programs are made more enjoyable for blind and low-vision viewers with the addition of a soundtrack that describes the key visual elements essential to the story line.

In the 1990s, the National Federation of the Blind, based in Baltimore, Maryland, launched its Newsline program. Daily papers were uploaded into a central computer each morning, and subscribers, by entering a password, could read the news by the simple use of their telephone. Long-distance charges were applicable in some cases.

The CNIB participated in this program for a few years, carrying the *Globe and Mail* along with some half-dozen American dailies. By 2000 the CNIB had facilitated Internet access to Canadian daily papers.

The Dayton M. Forman Memorial Award, established by the CNIB Library Board in January 1996, recognizes outstanding leadership in the advancement of library and information services for Canadians who are blind or visually impaired. It is offered in tribute to Dr. Dayton M. Forman, an exceptional humanitarian and longstanding CNIB volunteer who exemplified the leadership required to make a difference for over half a million visually impaired people across Canada.

In 2004, the award was presented to VoicePrint, which had become the world's largest service of its kind.

DIGITAL TECHNOLOGY

If records and cassettes are considered the first two generations of the talking book, in the 1990s digital technology became the third.

The Tower of Babel approach to audio books among nations may be about to end. This exciting and progressive development became possible with the formulation of an international standard known as the DAISY/NISO. Stated simply, digital books of the future will have one common standard allowing for production in either braille or audio format, regardless of the source. Today, blind readers have access to less than 3 percent of published material. New developments will hopefully mean that that information gap will close, as more books and magazines become available, in a timely manner, to blind readers.

The so-called DAISY CD has a capacity of forty hours or more of

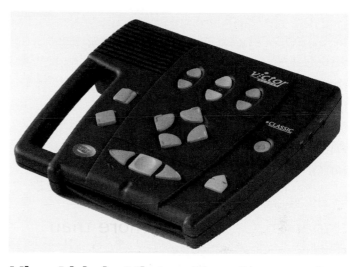

VisuAide's Victor Reader reads talking books recorded in digital format, making it much easier to navigate through a book.

audio recording, in contrast to seventy minutes on a commercial CD. There is general agreement that this is only an interim step in the evolution of the digital library.

Through Internet access and sophisticated access devices such as scanners, software for voice, or electronic braille, the well-trained blind library user will discover an entirely new world of lifelong learning and leisure reading. Downloaded from the Internet, current software makes it possible to have three or four full-length, professionally recorded audio books on one compact disc. However, Internet use has also raised a whole new set of legal and ethical copyright issues on a global scale.

The good news is that for the majority of blind Canadians, the information gap is closing rapidly.

Not so for the developing world. If anything, the gap is widening.

From the creativity and foresight of Thomas Edison to the genius of Bill Gates, the twenty-first century may yet belong to blindness and literacy.

CHAPTER 5
Blindness Prevention:
The Silent Paradox

According to the United Nations' World Health Organization, 150 million people around the globe have some kind of visual disability. (The number varies according to the source, and other organizations put that number as high as 180 million.) Of those, approximately 45 million are considered blind. And here's a number that's both shocking and sad: Sight Savers, an international blindness relief organization based in the U.K., says 80 percent of those people did not have to become blind. Worldwide, there are nearly 36 million people, more than the population of Canada, whose blindness would be considered preventable or curable.

Some people became blind because they did not have access to adequate medical care, including surgery and medication. Cataracts, a clouding of the eye's natural lens, are the leading cause of blindness around the world; an estimated 17 million people are blind because of them. And yet, the surgery to correct the condition is simple and relatively painless with a reported 90 percent success rate. Unfortunately, to many of those who need it, it just isn't available.

The second leading cause of blindness around the world is primary glaucoma, generally caused by an increase in pressure within the eye. In 2000, an estimated 6.7 million people were blind because of it, although prescribed eye drops in most cases can reduce the pressure and prevent vision loss. (Painless and symptomless in the early stages, glaucoma is called the silent thief of sight. In developed countries, like Canada, fewer than 50 percent of those who have it are aware of their disease. Detecting glaucoma is one reason why regular eye examinations are essential to vision health.)

Other contributing factors to preventable blindness include unsanitary living conditions, poor nutrition and hygiene, lack of sanitation facilities and clean water, and illiteracy. Not surprisingly, people at the highest risk for blindness live in developing countries, and were it not for a much lower life expectancy and high infant mortality rates in these soci-eties, the blindness figures would be considerably higher.

Despite massive efforts in public health, coordinated efforts by eye care professionals, and the allocation of hundreds of millions of dollars annually, blindness prevention remains an elusive objective as the numbers continue to climb. Vision 20-20, a global program to eliminate preventable blindness by the year 2020, is making a courageous and commendable effort, but the clock is counting down relentlessly and quickly.

In 2003, the CNIB reported 104,476 registered clients. However, a 1991 post-censal survey by Statistics Canada found 635,000 Canadians who identified themselves as having a significant level of vision loss that, even when wearing eyeglasses, affects their daily living. Many people are reluctant to identify themselves as having a visual impairment. Clearly, many Canadians who could benefit from the services of the CNIB and other agencies are not seeking out the assistance or are not aware that it exists. Of the 635,000 people who self-identified as blind or with low vision, 30,000 were children aged fourteen years and under.

People who are considered blind, or who have little or no light perception, make up less than 10 percent of those at risk. (In the public mind therefore, it is often confusing to determine the level of visual acuity or "sight" a person has.)

Myths like eye transplants remain in the realm of science fiction. An amusing anecdote on visual acuity and the difficulty to measure it was offered by Billy, a severely visually impaired boy in Winnipeg who, when asked by the eye care specialist, "How far can you see?", replied, "I don't know. How far is the sun?"

These limited paragraphs in no way attempt to chronicle the topic of blindness prevention or eye health. Entire libraries exist on the medical, social, psychological, and physiological causes of blindness as well as on its treatment and prevention. The purpose here is to report briefly on the role the CNIB played in vision health and blindness prevention since its founding, because the second of its two founding objectives was to prevent blindness.

In 1918, as soon as the organization was up and running, Irene Ewing, of Pike River, Quebec, was offered a one-year contract at $100 per month to work on blindness prevention. Ewing's early employment demonstrated the high priority the young institute was placing on eye health care. While it is not known now whether Ewing was a nurse, the CNIB has employed qualified nurses in the field of eye services throughout much of its history, and still does. In Quebec, however, the two rehabilitation centres adopted a different approach and today employ optometrists.

The CNIB's first honorary ophthalmologist, Dr. J.M. MacCallum, was also appointed in 1918. His role was to provide an authoritative opinion on the eye conditions of potential clients seeking rehabilitation from the institute. With the development and growth of programs offered by the CNIB, the need for an ophthalmological consultant to assist with the development and promotion of blindness prevention, research, and rehabilitation activities became obvious, and the position of consultant ophthalmologist was established.

Since 1918, nine prominent ophthalmologists have held the position, ending with Dr. G.A. Thompson, who, after his retirement in 1980, was never replaced.

However, in a major report commissioned by Managing Director Euclid Herie in 1984, author Charlene Muller, coordinator of blindness prevention, wrote:

> The necessity for a national consultant ophthalmologist has never been demonstrated more strongly than in the absence of the position. Without a consultant, the Institute is at the mercy of conflicting opinions from professional disciplines, the media do not view the CNIB as a reliable source of information in the blindness prevention areas, and above all, blindness prevention initiatives have suffered without professional direction and support.

The report recommended that a national consultant ophthalmologist be appointed, but this was not done.

In 1922, the CNIB partnered with such groups as the Red Cross, the Workmen's Compensation Boards, the International Order of Foresters, women's groups, and public health departments to distribute educational literature, known as propaganda, on eye health and blindness prevention.

At about the same time, generations of visually impaired students attended what became known as sight saving classes. (Blind students, or those nearly blind, attended the schools for the blind.) Only within the last decades of the twentieth century did educators come to believe that a student with impaired vision should use his residual vision to learn. From the early to mid-twentieth century, sight saving classes were designed for students whose vision was impaired and for whom it was believed that attempts to use residual vision came at the expense of losing it. Educational materials were dominated by texts featuring sight-saving methods.

Early educators believed that reading braille by sight "would be

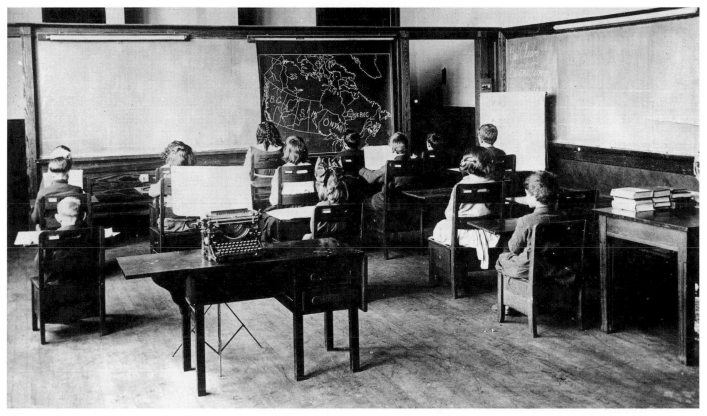

A sight saving class at Orde Street School in Toronto, 1924.

decidedly dangerous to students' vision and would very much lessen their reading abilities," as M.E. Frampton says in the 1936 work "The Training of Partially-Sighted Children in a School for the Blind." Students were reprimanded for using their vision. Braille-teaching materials included warning statements to educators, stating that students with vision impairments should never be allowed to read braille visually. Students who persisted in using vision to read were often blindfolded or required to wear high collars that made it impossible to use their eyesight.

This ideology held well into the second half of the century. Then, in 1969, school systems began to allow the use of residual vision following an American study by Natalie Barraga. Barraga's daughter was being taught braille at a school for the blind, but she tended to use her vision to read the braille pages. Barraga reasoned that if her daughter could read poor-contrast dots, then she could read high-contrast print Barraga's studies greatly influenced the field to encourage students to use their vision whenever possible.

The attitude still prevails among some parents and teachers, who don't seem to understand that print and braille are not competing and no harm will come from learning both.

The merit of sight saving classes is debatable. Exactly why placing students with serious visual impairments into designated classrooms was genuinely believed to somehow save their sight by its conservation and protection remains a mystery. The truth is that if a student had some kind of eye disease, sight saving classes alone were not the answer to vision health. Practically speaking, however, while this

practice separated visually impaired students from their peers, these children with special needs were at least in a public school and living at home with their families as opposed to being institutionalized for up to twelve years.

In 1961 the CNIB launched the Wise Owl Club of Canada, a blindness prevention program focusing on workplace safety. Within a decade, almost five thousand awards for eye safety had been presented to workers whose sight had been protected by safety

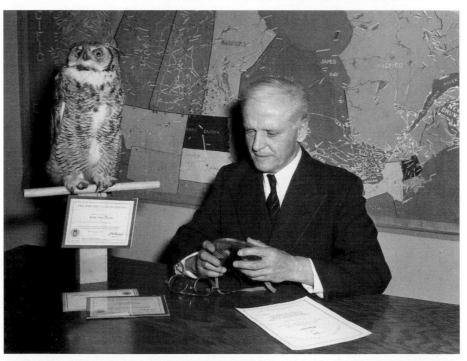

Edwin Baker launches the Wise Owl Club of Canada, 1961.

glasses or other eye wear during an on-the-job incident that could have resulted in an eye injury. As part of the program, CNIB staff also gave safety talks to mine and factory workers across Canada.

Other CNIB awareness programs included reaching out to schoolchildren using the Disney character Jiminy Cricket and starting public awareness and education campaigns on leading causes of blindness, such as glaucoma and diabetes.

The CNIB's National Council formalized its role in blindness prevention in 1923 when it appointed a Blindness Prevention committee. Almost immediately, the committee launched a major effort to eliminate blindness at birth from a condition known as *ophthalmia neonatorum* (acute conjunctivitis) or baby sore eyes, as it was colloquially called. This eye infection occurred in about 28 percent of infants born to mothers with venereal diseases and, if untreated, could cause blindness. From about the 1880s it had been known that a solution of silver nitrate applied to baby's eyes immediately after birth could prevent this type of blindness.

The CNIB applied pressure to the federal government and the provincial departments of health to insist that the treatment be legislated or in some way regulated. Some twenty years would pass before uniform application of the treatment eliminated the condition. These were early days in the understanding and application of public health measures and epidemiology.

Today, in most parts of Canada, silver nitrate is no longer used, but newborns' eyes are routinely treated with an antibiotic such as erythromycin as a precautionary measure.

TRACHOMA

Trachoma is another of the world's leading causes of preventable blindness. It's caused by the bacterium *Chlamydia trachomatis*, which can be spread easily by hands, clothing, or flies that have come in contact with discharge from the eyes or nose of an infected person. An infected mother may unknowingly pass the condition along to her baby simply by wiping his eyes with her scarf. The disease generally occurs in poor countries where people have limited access to clean water and good health care.

In Canada, British soldiers garrisoned in Quebec and Ontario in the mid-1850s are thought to have brought the infection with them from Britain. Later, settlers and explorers coming from the United States and elsewhere may also have been carriers of the disease.

The Canadian government, alarmed by the rapid spread of trachoma, amended the Immigration Act in 1902 prohibiting the entry of people known to be infected. This provision remained in force for at least seventy years.

Epidemics among native populations and in northern communities were rampant. In the 1930s, one clinic in Saskatchewan reported 245 active cases, 166 in children and teens under nineteen years of age. A Native reserve in southern Alberta reported more than one thousand active cases.

In 1931, the CNIB asked the federal government's Department of Indian Affairs to conduct a study on the incidence of trachoma among Native people.

Through public health measures such as improved sanitation and hygiene, education, and antibiotics, which the CNIB lobbied for, particularly in northern Canada, the disease has virtually been eliminated in North America. The CNIB 2003 client statistics pamphlet did not list trachoma as a diagnosis that would bring new clients to the organization.

Diphtheria, typhoid, smallpox, German measles, scarlet fever, and tuberculosis eventually were either eliminated or reduced significantly by inoculation programs, public health programs, and remedial medical treatment. Early diagnosis and more points of entry into the health system, combined with heightened professional knowledge and training, account for Canada's excellent record in blindness prevention.

However, sports injuries, home or automobile accidents, and substance abuse, such as glue sniffing, inhaling gasoline fumes, or drinking toxic substances such as methyl alcohol, can all cause blindness that in some cases would have been preventable. Genetic counselling, an emerging resource, may also play a role in blindness prevention.

BLINDNESS PREVENTION IN THE NORTH

One of the most fascinating chapters in the CNIB's role in blindness prevention took place in 1945 when three intrepid eye care workers took up the challenge of the Eastern Arctic Eye Patrols, embarking on a sixteen-thousand-kilometre trip through icy northern waters aboard the RMS *Nascopie*, a ship belonging to the Hudson's Bay Company.

The three had diverse professional expertise: Dr. Walter Crewson was an ophthalmologist, Margaret Moeller was a nurse and secretary of Blindness Prevention with the CNIB eye service, and Flight Lieutenant A.H. Tweedle was an optometrist and a former member of the Royal Canadian Air Force.

The eye care team held eye clinics, whenever possible at hospitals such as the one at Chesterfield Inlet on the west coast of Hudson Bay and Pangnirtung at the southeast of Baffin Island. The team also treated those requiring surgical procedures, although follow-up care was left in the capable hands of the resident physician and nurses.

This Snellen eye chart, printed with Inuit syllabics, was used in the early Eastern Arctic Eye Patrols sponsored by the CNIB.

125

Where such facilities were not available, the team used the *Nascopie*'s tiny dispensary. Imagine performing eye surgery aboard a turn-of-the-century ship, roiling in Arctic waters in a three-by-three-metre room with your patient and five observers. Dr. Crewson examined 208 Inuit, of whom 126 had normal eyes. He found seven totally blind individuals and others needing corrective lenses. In many cases the CNIB paid for eyeglasses, artificial eyes, and medicine. They performed procedures en route and then left their patients at the hospital at Pangnirtung for after-care. The *Nascopie* would then pick up the recovered Inuit on her next voyage and return them to their homes.

This was a major project, as Moeller noted: "It is quite an undertaking to arrange for operations and care for these people and especially so when the patient is the head of the family which means the removal of the patient, his family, dogs and household goods for a year at least."

The medical findings of the eye care team were interesting. On the whole, they found that the Inuit had healthy eyes. For the most part, any blindness seen on the 1945 trip was due to trauma — often due to rifle accidents.

Some patients related that their history of eye trouble had started as simple snow blindness. Various reports give descriptions of ingenious efforts at fashioning the perfect snow goggles — with mixed results.

John Baker, son of CNIB co-founder Edwin Baker, recalled how his father, a skilled woodworker, manufactured wooden and felt snow goggles that were distributed to Arctic residents.

In 1945, the federal department of Health and Welfare Canada was urged to set up two permanent eye-service units in the north to provide regular eye examinations and to help eradicate common eye diseases. Although the Eastern Arctic Eye Patrols were discontinued in 1954, the stage was set for the provision of ongoing, quality eye care.

The northernmost portion of Canada, bordering in part on the Arctic Ocean, comprises one third of Canada's land mass. By 1980, fewer than one hundred of the some fifty thousand residents in the entire area were registered

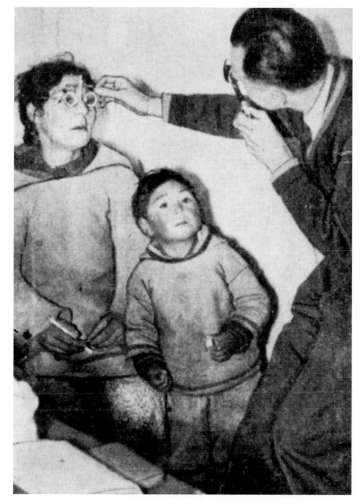

An Eye Patrol member examines the eyes of an Inuit woman.

with the CNIB, although it had been providing service to the area for many years, as this account from the first issue of *National News of the Blind*, from January 1936, reveals.

There is one blind person in Canada with whom the Institute is in touch only once a year. Each September, if all goes well, the little government steamer which makes a tour of the islands in the Arctic archipelago, calls in at Pangnirtung, a little port on the east shore of Baffinland. That is where Mrs. William Duval, blind Eskimo woman, lives. She is the only Eskimo woman on the register of the Institute and her residence is farther north than that of any other blind Canadian.... Braille books, home teaching or street car passes were not much use to Mrs. Duval but the Institute did send her a parcel containing a few small gifts — tobacco, needles, thread, candy. Although blind, Mrs. Duval is quite able to perform the two most essential duties required of Eskimo housewives — she can sew and cook … Proof of her skill at sewing came to the Institute in the form of a set of beautifully made Eskimo woman's summer clothes, a pair of seal-hide mucklucks and two seal-skin rugs. The sewing on these articles is … exquisitely done.

By 1982, the CNIB recognized that it needed to provide better services to this group of clients, many of whom live in isolated communities.

The discovery of a sizable number of cases of hereditary Retinitis pigmentosa in the community of Rae-Edzo, near Yellowknife, emphasized the need for services.

James Sanders, then executive director of the Alberta-NWT division, and Wendy Edey, service coordinator for northern Alberta, led teams of service personnel into the north. National Council endorsed the recommendation from the Alberta Board in 1982 and expanded the division to include the Northwest Territories. In 1986, Bill McKeown, executive director of the Alberta-NWT division, and CNIB Managing Director Euclid Herie were in Yellowknife on a sub-zero November day to open the new district office.

"It was like an Easter egg hunt as we had to locate pockets of money to finance an office," McKeown recalled. Prior to the opening of the office, CNIB teams made infrequent trips north, and clients were brought south to Edmonton or Calgary for training. McKeown put it best when he described how the services CNIB was providing its northernmost clients might not have been what they needed or wanted. "We were training them to cook with microwaves, ride fast transit systems, and navigate malls. What they really wanted, in many cases, was simply to learn how to cook caribou stew over an open fire."

In 1999, when Nunavut became a separate territory in the eastern Arctic, the Alberta-NWT division added it to its sphere of responsibility and name.

EYE BANKS

The Eye Bank began in 1955 as a joint effort of the Canadian Ophthalmological Society (COS) and the CNIB. Today, hospitals, service clubs, and universities are joining the effort with funding, research, and volunteer support. Thousands of Canadians are today enjoying excellent sight through the selfless actions of eye donors, people who agreed that at the time of their death their eyes could be used for medical purposes, including research, teaching, and transplantation of the cornea. According to Health Canada, 2,602 corneal transplants took place in 2000, with 3,269 people on waiting lists.

The COS strongly endorses the work of the eye banks that have been set up in various regions of Canada. These organizations speed the use of donated eyes, which must be removed not later than eight hours after death and used within forty-eight hours.

In 1963, however, for the first time in history, the Ontario division of the Eye Bank of Canada received eyes from a living blind person, Mrs. Oster, a resident of the CNIB's Edgewood Hall in Hamilton. The donation was described in the *National News of the Blind*.

"I thank God that they could do something with my poor old eyes

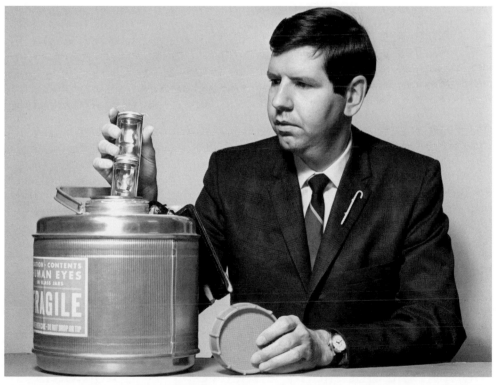

Claude Maurice of the Quebec Eye Bank, 1968.

which weren't any good to me," she said. "If I'd had any idea that my eyes could be of use to anybody, I'd have had this done long ago."

"The Bank was crazy to get them," noted W.K. Lawson, Hamilton field secretary, adding that Mrs. Oster's actions not only made history but also illustrated the urgent needs of the Eye Bank of Canada.

That same year, an eye bank was opened in Whitehorse, Yukon Territory. Anyone aged eighteen years or over can become a donor by signing the form on one's driving license or a form available from an eye bank.

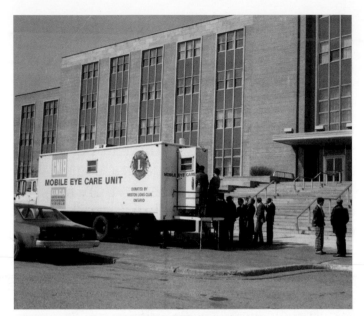

This Eye Van, donated by the Lions Club of Weston, Ontario, visited thousands of scattered towns and outposts throughout Newfoundland and Labrador.

MEDICAL MOBILE EYE CARE UNITS (EYE VANS)

In several major service centres, the CNIB offers low vision services to people who, while not considered blind, are vision impaired. Usually, services are provided in rooms equipped with high-tech devices such as closed-circuit television screen readers that enlarge print and low-tech devices such as the humble but highly effective magnifying glass.

The approach taken, and level of staffing provided, varies from one location to another. Usually, however, the service features a frontline nurse who assists clients in determining which devices best suit their needs, depending on their level of vision and what it is they want or need to do.

The nurses also provide important follow-up with clients if an optometrist or ophthalmologist has recommended or prescribed a specific treatment or technical device. One or both of these professionals may also attend at CNIB clinics where facilities allow.

Providing much higher visibility of the CNIB's role in low vision services were the Medical Mobile Eye Care Units (Eye Vans) that travelled the highways and byways of Ontario, Newfoundland, and Quebec for many years, bringing eye health care to remote regions.

In all three provinces, Lions Clubs were among the main financial contributors and logistical supporters.

In the 1980s, the service was discontinued in Quebec and Newfoundland because of funding issues and shifting priorities. And, like the closure of the residences, in Quebec and Newfoundland the decision to discontinue the service was unpopular and not understood by the communities affected.

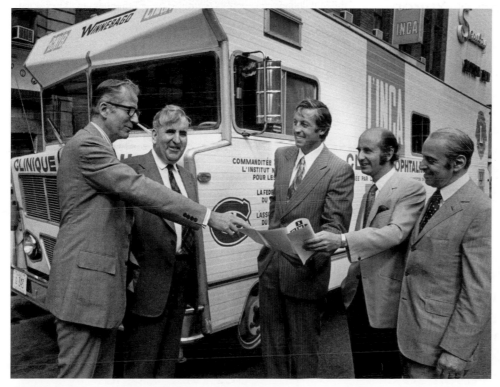

Hockey great Jean Beliveau, centre, of the Montreal Canadiens lends his support to the Eye Van in 1973.

But in Ontario, each year, from March to November, the Eye Van, a custom-made transport truck and 14.6-metre trailer containing state-of-the-art medical eye care equipment, brings the best in medical eye care to remote areas in northern Ontario where services are not available. Twenty ophthalmologists volunteer for one-week periods to examine, treat, and perform minor surgery on about five thousand patients each season. The doctors are assisted by two CNIB nurses. Clients served include people with serious eye problems or a family history of eye disease, children and seniors experiencing difficulties due to vision loss, patients with diabetes and glaucoma, and people unable to get a routine eye examination because there is no eye care professional in their area.

The Eye Van is not only about prevention and healing. Through the sponsorship of two pharmaceutical companies, Allergan Inc. and CIBA Vision Ophthalmics, special medical education programs are available for local doctors and nurses, and doctors and CNIB nurses travelling with the Eye Van also promote their service by speaking to community groups.

In 2000, a CNIB committee considered expanding the program into northern areas of western Canada, but neither the political will nor the funding could be found to mount and sustain such an ambitious and costly initiative. Further, public health policies and services have changed, as have government priorities.

Clearly, like the Technibus of 1993, the CNIB could not generate a higher profile "road show" than the Eye Van as it arrives in small, remote northern communities for its much anticipated annual visit. Townsfolk roll out the welcome mat and provide advance publicity and volunteers to ensure the success of the mobile clinic.

Conceived in 1971 by Ross Purse, then director of the CNIB's Ontario division, and Dr. William S. Hunter, chair of the Ontario Medical Association's Section on Ophthalmology, the Eye Van is an integral part of both organizations' Prevention of Blindness programs.

E.A. BAKER FOUNDATION

In 1962, in honour of the retirement of its most celebrated co-founder, the CNIB created a special foundation.

Its creation was recorded in the National Council minutes:

> In recognition of Colonel Baker's forty-two years of unrelenting and unsurpassed service in the alleviation of blindness, and in the hope that his name may forever be

perpetuated as an outstanding Canadian, the CNIB do establish a fund to be administered by this Council and to be known as the E.A. Baker Foundation for the Prevention of Blindness.

Close to $100,000 was donated from CNIB divisions and around the world to launch the foundation.

Today, the foundation annually awards fellowships for advanced post-graduate training in ophthalmic sub-specialties and provides grants of up to $40,000 to encourage new investigations that may lead to the prevention of blindness. More than $9 million has been given.

EYE CARE PROFESSIONALS

Any discussion of eye health care in Canada would be incomplete without a brief reference to the professionals in the field. It's well known that for decades the professions of optometry and ophthalmology have been unable to see eye to eye, so to speak, on the respective roles and areas of practice they each should perform in vision health. For example, before the policy change of 1986 and the SEE program, the CNIB would only accept a formal referral and the actual registration of a person as "blind" with an approved medical form that required the signature of an ophthalmologist. This meant that no other eye health practitioners could refer a patient to the CNIB, which was a major irritant for the optometrists. This public debate peaked during Robert Mercer's term as managing director. It's fair to say that the change in policy within the CNIB led to a major philosophical discussion before the decision was made that CNIB services would be offered without the requirement of a medical referral. In the minds of some, the issue of service referral remains an unanswered question.

At times these professional differences, some might say jealousies, have become public and the source of competing petitions before governments for legislated and regulated policies dealing with eye care.

The average Canadian patient, seeking good medical care, could not have cared less about the issues dividing the two groups. However, long waiting lists for surgery and remedial medical treatment had become a growing concern by the closing decades of the twentieth century.

In the 1980s, CNIB Managing Director Euclid Herie determined that better relations among the major stakeholders in Canada was essential, and after fifteen years of persistent trying, his efforts paid off.

In 1998, under the auspices of the E.A. Baker Foundation for the Prevention of Blindness, the CNIB hosted the National Consultation on the Crisis in Vision Loss. For the first time in decades, if ever, representatives from government, consumer and advocacy groups, health care professions, social services agencies, academia, and industry came together to identify the key issues and challenges associated with vision loss and to establish them on Canada's public health agenda.

At the close of the three-day conference, Ian Potter, assistant deputy minister of Health Canada, presented the participants with three years' significant funding to launch the Vision Health Coalition, which could well serve as a model for other nations facing similar issues. (Was this the CNIB's finest hour, sponsoring the forum that brought this result funded initially by the federal government? Not likely, but it was a historic first!)

Not until the 1990s was age-related macular degeneration (AMD) recognized as a leading cause of blindness, especially in people over fifty — a problem that was going largely untreated.

Macular degeneration causes loss of ability to see detail at any distance. It affects reading, driving, seeing faces, threading a needle, cutting your toenails, and a host of other activities. Smoking is the major controllable risk factor, and although there are no treatments that can restore vision lost through macular degeneration, a diet rich in vegetables and fruits and specially formulated vitamin and mineral combinations can slow the progression in about 25 percent of cases of the more common "dry" form. In the "wet" form, which makes up about 10 percent of AMD, a small percentage of patients have experienced stabilization of their conditions through a surgical treatment pioneered in Canada.

The procedure involves the injection of a dye called Visudyne, developed in Vancouver, followed by application by a cold laser beam, all performed by an ophthalmologist. The CNIB has worked with the ophthalmological community in securing provincial health coverage of the procedure.

In 2002, the CNIB undertook a major national awareness initiative, holding public forums on AMD in fourteen Canadian cities. An ophthalmologist explained the medical aspects of the condition, a CNIB vision rehabilitation specialist described how a vision assessment and low vision service aids could help, and a person with macular degeneration talked about the emotional impact and coping strategies.

The sessions' popularity was beyond the organizers' expectations. Many hundreds of people, most of them middle aged or elderly, drove great distances to attend, and the first few sessions were standing room only. For later sessions in the series, larger rooms were booked. In partnership with Novartis Ophthalmics, the CNIB produced public service announcements and a documen-tary on macular degeneration featuring actor Mary Walsh, who has a form of the condition.

The CNIB continues its educational campaign about AMD through public meetings, media events, and website information, and staff in Ottawa and provincial capitals continue their efforts to educate politicians and public servants about the need for coverage of the cost of functional vision assessments and treatments.

The CNIB was also a founding member of the AMD Alliance International, a nonprofit coalition of the world's leading vision and seniors' organizations represented in twenty-one countries. As an awareness and public education organization, it has its work cut out for it. Although eighty thousand Canadians are diagnosed with macular degeneration each year, only 1 percent of Canadians can identify it as the leading cause of vision loss in this country.

Longer life expectancy and the aging process account for the fact that 50 percent of the CNIB's newly registered clients in 2003 had been diagnosed with AMD, compared to 6.8 percent who had become visually impaired because of complications from diabetes.

From that first 1918 letter to Irene Ewing to the creation of the E.A. Baker Foundation for the Prevention of Blindness in 1962 to the National Consultation on the Crisis in Vision Loss of 1998, the CNIB has funded, advocated, and supported improved vision health and blindness prevention in Canada, including financial and active support for such projects as Vision 20-20 — and this will continue into the future.

Events such as World Sight Day, held on Parliament Hill in Ottawa in October 2003, bring together a consortium of concerned organizations to create awareness and carry out the CNIB's mandate as the founders had envisioned it.

For the CNIB, the challenge is to find the balance between providing service for clients and preventing blindness so fewer Canadians have to become clients. A daunting paradox.

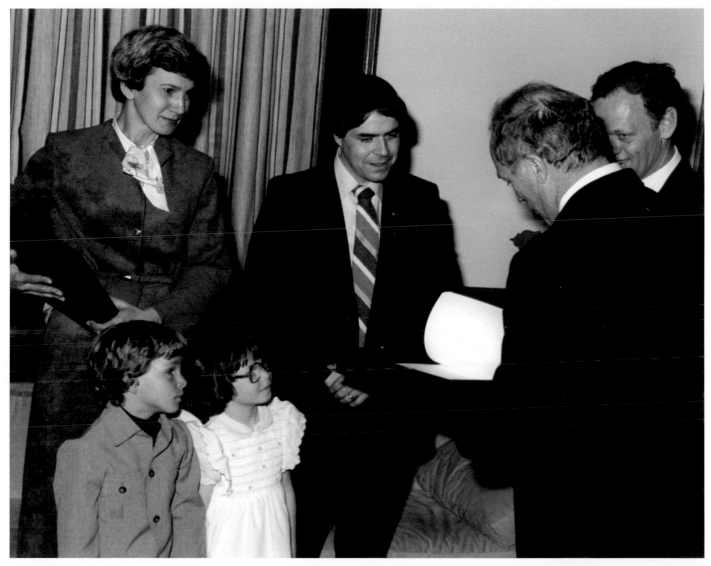

Darleen Bogart, chair of the CNIB National Library Division board, and Robert Mercer, managing director, assisted by two young clients, Mario Miville from Quebec and Valerie Hastings from Regina, present Prime Minister Pierre Trudeau with a braille version of the amendments to the Canadian Constitution on April 17, 1982. Looking on is Justice Minister Jean Chrétien.

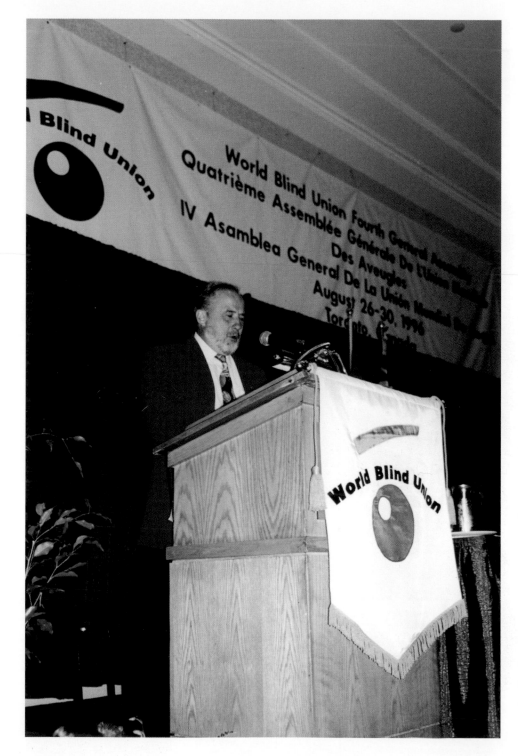

LEFT: Euclid Herie accepts the presidency of the World Blind Union at the fourth general assembly in Toronto, 1996.

FACING PAGE: Euclid Herie (left) receives the Order of Canada from Governor General Romeo Leblanc, 1997.

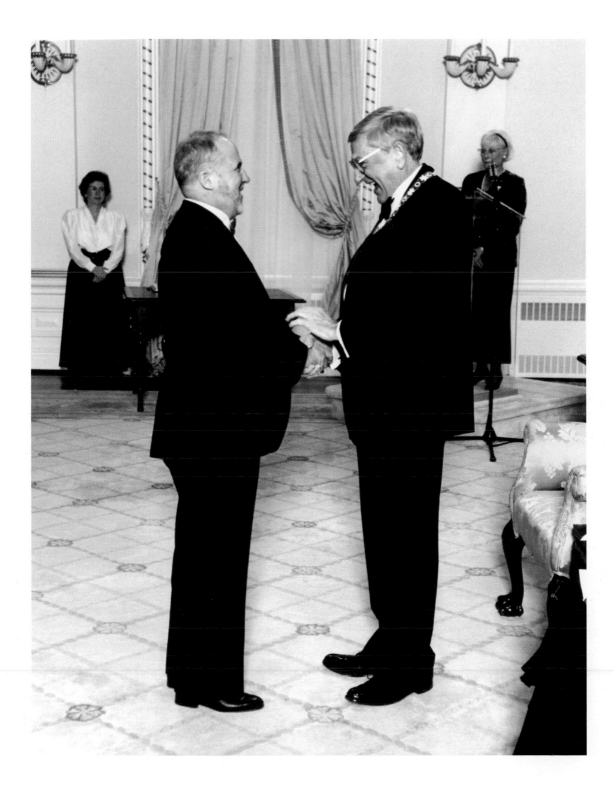

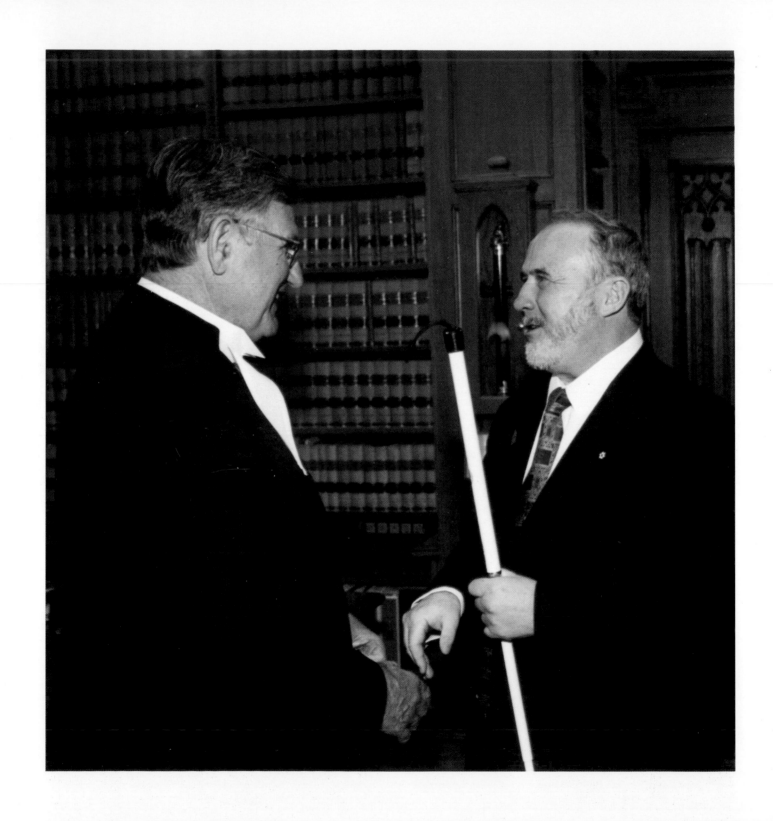

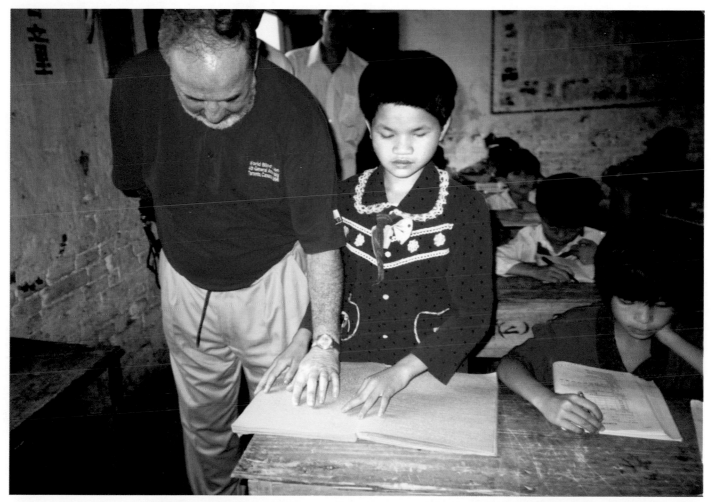

ABOVE: On a 1998 visit to China, Euclid Herie visited the Fushan School, where he met young Pan Xing Lang, who showed him Mandarin braille.

FACING PAGE: Speaker of the House of Commons Gilbert Parent (left) welcomes Euclid Herie to Parliament Hill on the occasion of the CNIB's eightieth anniversary, 1998.

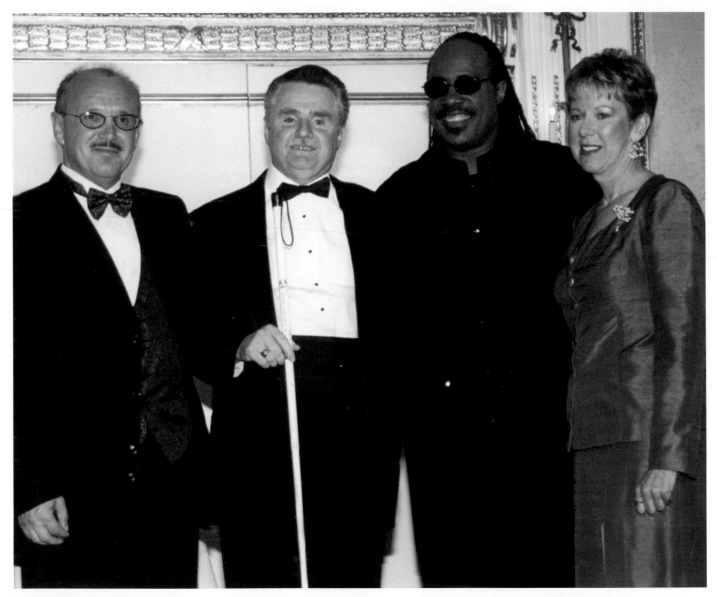

(Left to right) CEO Paul Wahl of SAP America, CNIB Vice-President James Sanders, musician Stevie Wonder, and CNIB Director of Human Resources Mary Ann Roscoe at the presentation of the SAP/Stevie Wonder Award to the CNIB as a role model organization, 1998.

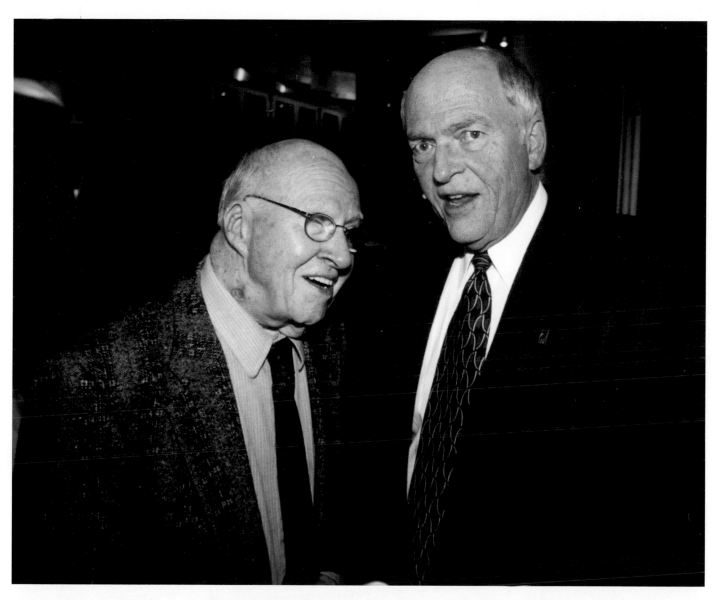

Long-time CNIB public relations director Paul O'Neill (left) is congratulated by board chair Gary Homer on receiving the Grace Worts Award for outstanding employee service, 1999.

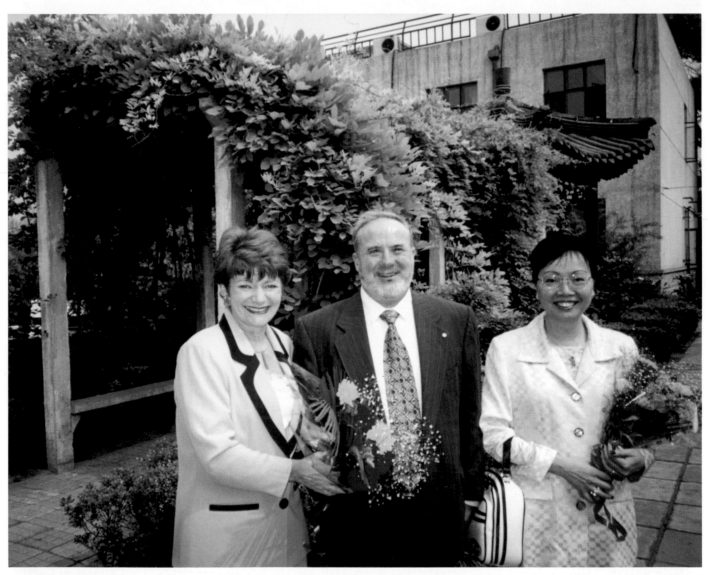

(Left to right) CNIB Corporate Secretary Barbara Marjeram, Euclid Herie, and Grace Chan, executive director of the Hong Kong Society for the Blind, 1999.

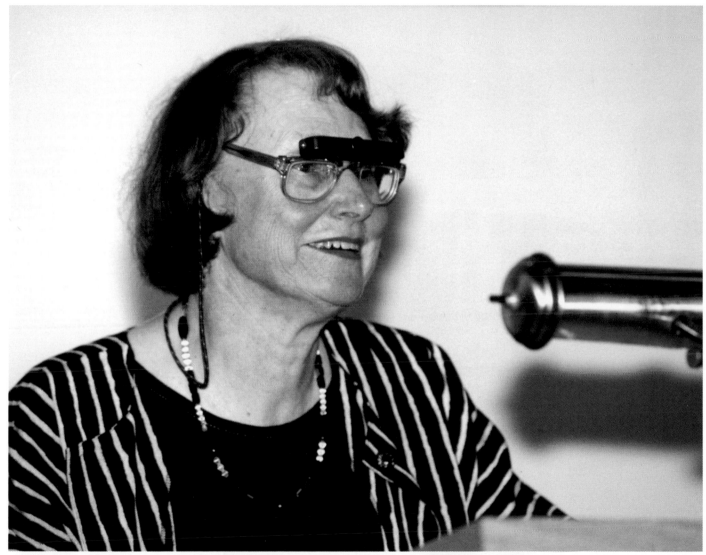

Frances Cutler of Ottawa, CNIB chair from 2000 to 2003.

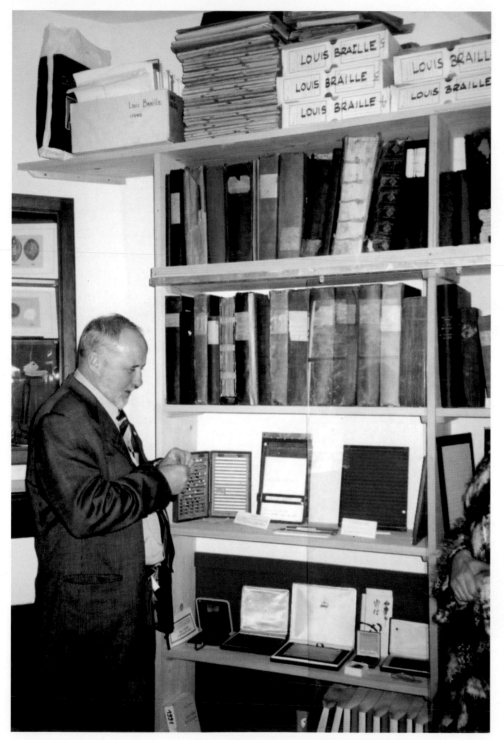

LEFT: Euclid Herie, who led the charge to preserve Louis Braille's birthplace in Coupvray, France, visits the museum, 2001.

FACING PAGE: CNIB client Timothy Peters, ten, explores the world's first Children's Discovery Portal, sponsored by Microsoft Canada, as CNIB President Jim Sanders, Microsoft Chairman and Chief Software Architect Bill Gates, and CNIB President Emeritus Euclid Herie respond to questions from the media.

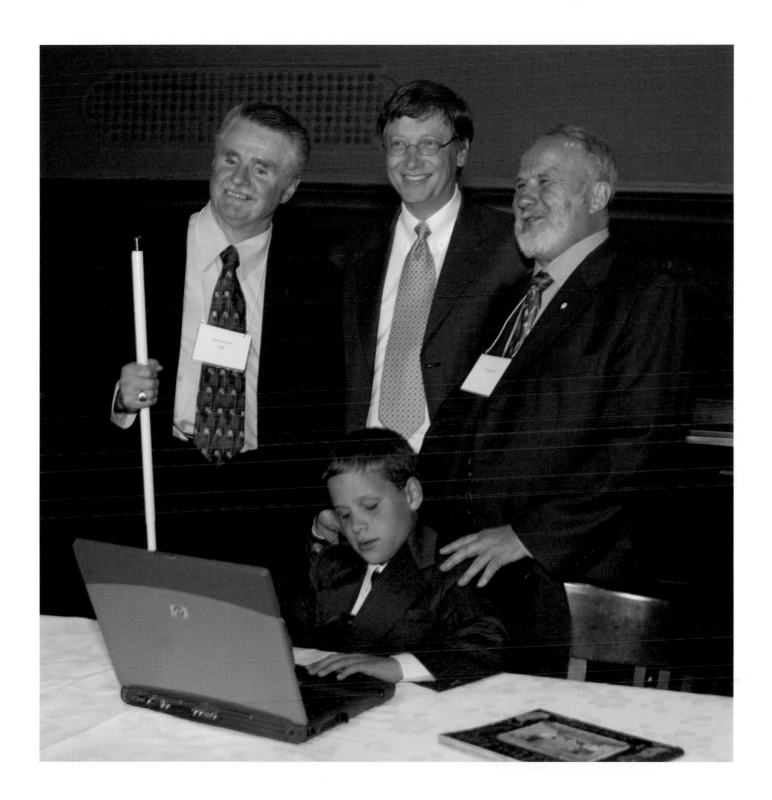

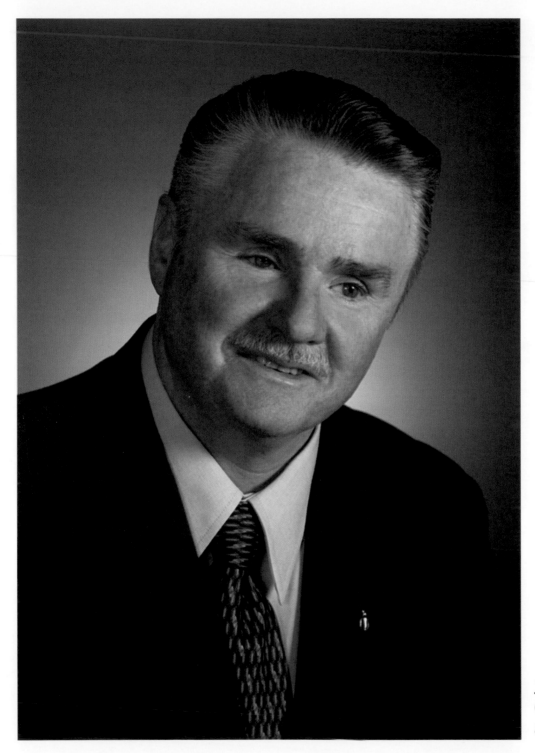

James Sanders,
CNIB president
and CEO.

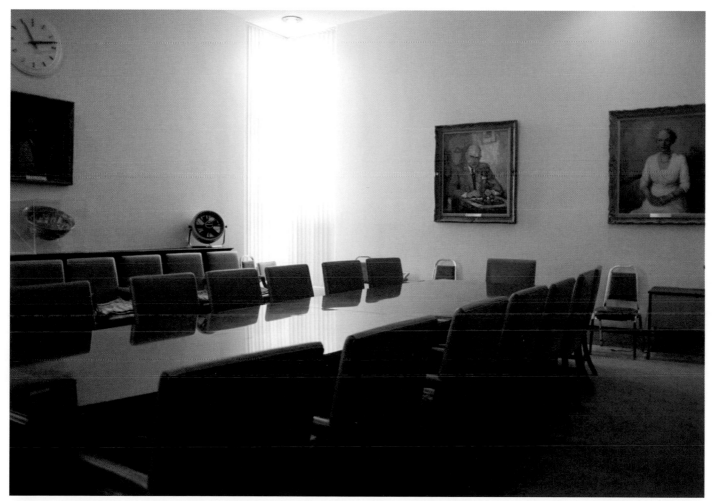

The CNIB boardroom, with portraits of Lieutenant-Colonel Edwin Baker, Lewis Wood, and Lady Kemp.

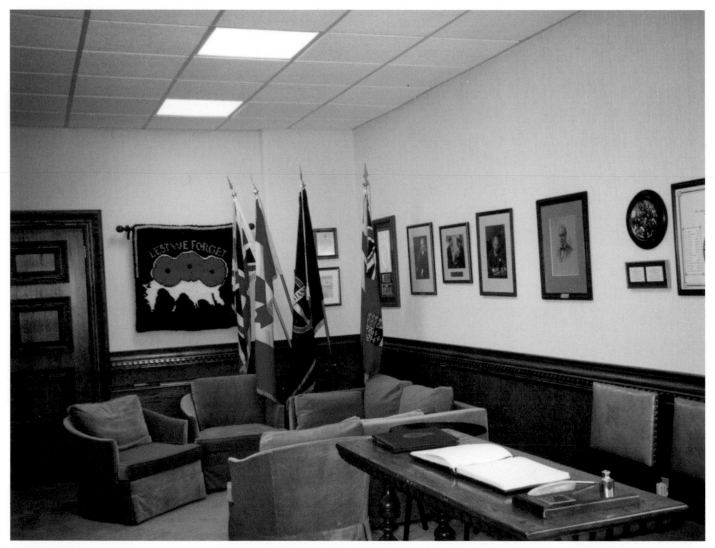

The Sir Arthur Pearson Association Lounge at BakerWood, 1929 Bayview Avenue, Toronto.

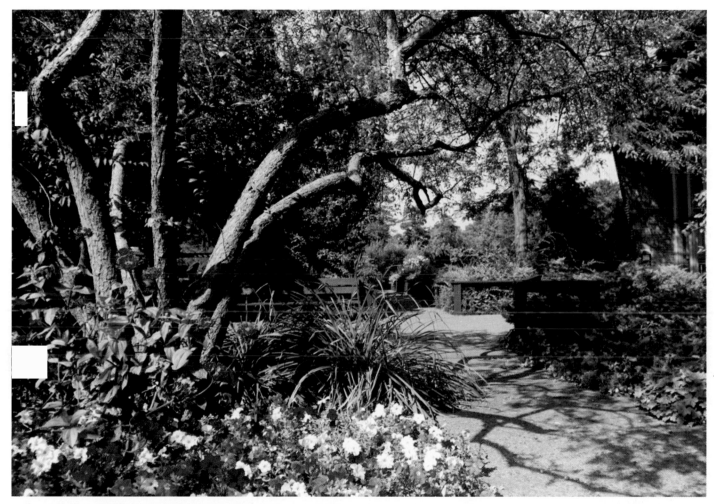

The beautiful Fragrant Garden at BakerWood in Toronto, which served as a model for others around the world.

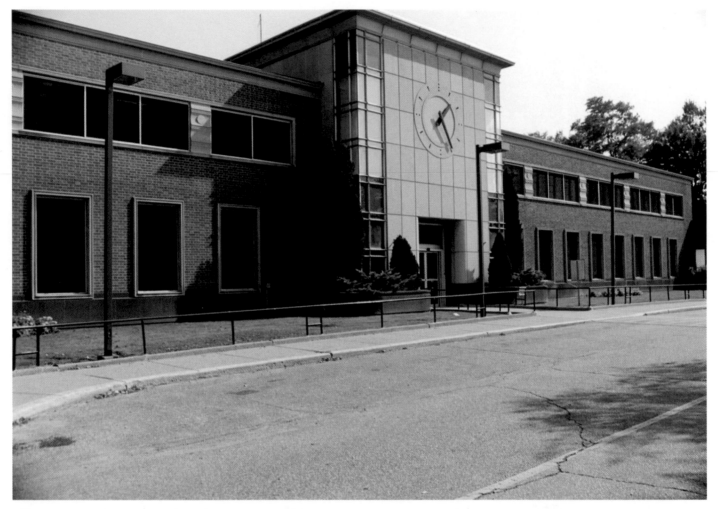

The facade at 1929 Bayview Avenue in 2001, showing the clock tower. The building was demolished in 2002.

CHAPTER 6
Unsung Heroes: Home Teachers

In an undated paper thought to have been written in about 1956, Margaret Liggett describes the early days of her work as a CNIB home teacher:

> For more than 30 years, I served on the staff of The Canadian National Institute for the Blind as home teacher in Saskatchewan: or, as I often called myself, travelling teacher. This self-bestowed title was assumed because so many reporters referred to me in news items as 'the teacher from the home for the blind.' Actually, my duty was to visit homes of people who lost their sight in adult life. Being past student age, these citizens are not eligible to attend government schools provided for blind children.
>
> A home teacher's prospective pupil may

live in an isolated corner of the province. If so, reaching his home generally involved a trip on a mixed train which stopped at every station to load and unload heavy freight and live stock. This was followed by a long, rough ride behind horses. This mode of travel allows ample time for contemplation of one's immediate future. For the next few weeks I would be living with some family of whom I knew nothing; confronted with the task of teaching some member of that circle the art of living in a new world of darkness.

In a 1978 interview, Lucille Sellinger (née Savoy) explained how she arrived in Regina just as Liggett, whom she described as a legend, was retiring. Sellinger, who had been trained as a home teacher in Toronto in 1952, described some of Liggett's adventures as a home teacher, including being confined to a student's home for six weeks when a snowstorm made travel impossible.

For us now to appreciate fully the accomplishments of the home teachers of the early part of the twentieth century, we must revisit them in their geographic context.

VAST TERRITORIES

The three western Canadian provinces of Manitoba, Saskatchewan, and Alberta comprise the Prairies. Manitoba joined Confederation in 1870, and Saskatchewan and Alberta followed thirty-five years later in 1905.

Before that, Saskatchewan and Alberta had been part of an immense tract of land known as the Northwest Territories. The area stretched west from the Red River settlement (later the site of the city of Winnipeg at the joining of the Red and Assiniboine rivers) to Calgary, Alberta, nestled in the foothills of the Canadian Rocky Mountains. This is a distance of more than sixteen hundred kilometres running more or less parallel to the Canada–United States border.

To the north, the territory stretched to the Arctic Circle. In

1905, the two provinces had been carved out of the southern half of the territory, and the remainder, one-third of Canada's land mass of 9 million square kilometres, formed the Western Arctic and the Eastern Arctic, administered from Ottawa until 1967, when Yellowknife became the territorial capital. In 1999, the Northwest Territories was divided, creating the Northwest Territories in the west and Nunavut in the east, each with its own government.

Imagine, then, the fledgling Canadian National Institute for the Blind taking on the enormous task of identifying and serving blind people scattered within this massive geographic area. Not only that, but the blind people were hidden on remote farms, small hamlets in the south, and isolated hunting and fishing encampments in the far north. From the perspective of the jet and satellite age, the transportation and communication barriers seem to have been insurmountable.

Nevertheless, starting in 1920, home teachers, field men, and later nursing and related eye health care workers ventured out across the great land in all weathers, from blistering summer heat to the freezing rains of late winter. They travelled by whatever means were available to them: on foot, by horse and buggy, on steam trains, and eventually, after roads were expanded, by motor car. In the north, dog sleds and canoes were the conveyances of choice.

The features of British Columbia, with its Pacific Island archipelago and towering mountain ranges, and the Yukon territory to the north presented a different set of challenges to expanding services to blind residents.

For the intrepid Margaret Liggett, who joined the CNIB as a home teacher in 1921, the path was rough but the rewards were many.

"Before my Saskatchewan teaching schedule could be planned, prospective pupils must be located," she wrote. "So a year was spent on a survey, hunting for blind citizens and learning their needs. Saskatchewan boasted neither bus nor air travel and good highways were rare."

Prairie folk are a tough and self-reliant lot, but Liggett helped many of them — men, women, and children — make the adjustment to vision loss by teaching them new skills and new ways of doing familiar things.

Visually impaired herself, Liggett also provided encouragement and understanding. In her brief memoir, Liggett describes some of her more memorable experiences with her Saskatchewan clients.

A few years after the move to Candle Lake, Mrs. Stephens developed eye trouble which ultimately culminated in blindness. An eye specialist, knowing that no treatment could help, sent her to the CNIB office in Regina where arrangements were made for her to have lessons at home.

The duties of a pioneer home teacher in an ever expanding province had often taken me to newly-settled farming districts yet this request in 1941 was the first to come from the margin of that great beyond where agriculture is not even the dream of the future.

Meath Park was the closest railway point and could be reached from Prince Albert by CPR [Canadian Pacific Railway] three times a week. Mail was taken to Candle Lake from Meath Park every Saturday and the mail carrier had room for one passenger. A letter had been written to Mrs. Stephens saying that I would arrive on the first September mail.

So while I boarded Friday's train in Prince Albert, Mr. Stephens stood on the trail watching for the mail carrier on his way to Meath Park. Having arranged for my coming, he sent me verbal instructions to get myself something to eat on the thirty mile drive. The mail carrier hunted me up that evening in Meath Park. He took my baggage checks as everything must be loaded to insure an early start next morning. Gravelled roads were increasing and most rural mail was being delivered by car. By morning it was raining heavily. As I waited in the Meath Park Hotel, I wondered if the mud would be so deep that our car would skid off the road. To my surprise the mailman pulled up in a horse-drawn, canvas-covered vehicle.

For the first eight miles we passed small farms newly cleared of bush, then entered the dense forest. Gloomy, wet pine-scented air creates an appetite, and I began speculating about the approaching meal. It seemed likely that we would stop at some half-breed home for dinner. Suddenly, the driver remarked that having passed the settlement we would see no more signs of human life until towards evening. Our destination would not be reached until after dark. That seemed a long time to fast.

At noon we halted. The driver unhitched and fed the horses then produced our dinner. Instead of delivering Mr. Stephens' message, he had asked a Meath Park friend to pack a nice lunch for me. Don't ask me how this experienced woodsman lit a fire in the rain, boiled water and made tea. I know he did it.

My mission to Candle Lake was to give Mrs. Stephens an opportunity to learn Braille, typing, handicrafts and adjustment to blindness. But life there was so different from any former experience that I probably learned more than I taught … Mrs. Stephens finished her lessons early in October…. A home teacher usually experiences either regret or satisfaction when leaving a pupil. On the drive back to Meath Park, I was conscious of both emotions. Knowledge that CNIB Braille library books find their way into lonely homes like the one I had just left was heart warming. It was also pleasant to think of the baby basket which Mrs. Stephens was making for an infant grandson. But what home teacher, meditating on the material needs of some pupil, has not yearned for a millionaire's bank account? Handicrafts in Candle Lake could not be turned into remunerative channels, for where there is no population, there is no market.

Liggett continued her career with the CNIB until her retirement. In 1955 she was awarded a gold medal and honorary life membership in the Canadian Council of the Blind (CCB) in recognition of her pioneering work as a home teacher. A framed tribute to her hanging in the CNIB Regina office reads, in part:

In 1920 The Canadian National Institute for the Blind organized its first home teacher's course. In 1921 you responded to the call, entering a field which, at that time, was unexplored and undeveloped in Canada. For thirty-two years you travelled the length and breadth of your province — from the open, wind-swept prairies of the South to the parkland and bush country of the North; from thriving urban communities to remote homesteads; always with one purpose uppermost in your mind — to give blind people the instruction, encouragement and inspiration which would help them in their struggle to adjust to their loss of sight. Your all-encompassing love of humanity knew no barriers of race, creed, colour or economic conditions. Whenever there

came a call for help,
your response was
always the same —
"Here am I, send me."

Liggett died in 1966.

HISTORY OF HOME TEACHING

The concept of providing blind people with instruction in the familiar surroundings of their own homes is thought to have begun in nineteenth-century England when William Moon, creator of a specialized system of raised type, arranged for books, mainly of a Biblical nature, to be distributed among newly blinded adults. In 1855, the Society for Supplying Home Teachers and Books in Moon Type was founded in London. The first teacher employed by the Society was a blind man who in the course of 20 years taught 402 blind people to read. But although Dr. Moon and others believed that in general blind people made better teachers of the blind than sighted people because of their ability to inspire and motivate, the home teaching movement in England did not continue the prac-

tice of employing blind teachers because it was felt that sighted teachers could travel about more cheaply and easily.

The home teaching movement spread throughout Great Britain and then reached North American shores. Sir Frederick Fraser, who was for many years superintendent of the School for the Blind in Halifax, is credited with offering the first home teaching programs in Canada during the 1890s. Although his primary responsibility was to the blind schoolchildren, he did feel concern for the adult blind — especially those who lost their sight in their later years. To meet the needs of this group, Sir Frederick established the School Extension Service.

Sir Frederick was adamant in his belief that a blind person who had experienced and overcome his handicap would be the most help to newly blinded adults, and it was from the graduates of the Halifax School that he chose Canada's first home teacher for the adult blind.

Her name was Una Legg, and she was sent, following her graduation from the Halifax School, to a training school in London, England, where she studied massage and hairdressing. On her return to Canada in 1893, she began her work by seeking out the blind and giving them instruction in their homes. In a letter, the versatile Ms. Legg described what she did and how she did it:

I taught the work for about seven years. Their ages ran from twenty-five to sixty-five. The ones who could learn Braille easily I taught Braille, but others I taught the Moon system. The women I taught knitting, crochet, bead work, shampooing and some the auto-harp. Of course I stayed at the homes of the students, if that were convenient, and if not, I boarded near by. I taught one old gentleman of sixty-five, an old American soldier, who was staying with his daughter at St. Andrew's. He later went to a soldier's home in Maine and taught Braille to some blind men there. He was my star

pupil. Of course the school paid my travelling expenses and my salary was five dollars a month.

By 1919, the home teaching program offered by the Halifax School for the Blind was in serious financial difficulty, and this proved to be where the paths of the CNIB and the school crossed. This excerpt from the fiftieth annual report of the board of managers and the superintendent of the Halifax School for the Blind in 1920 describes how the two organizations came to pool their resources:

Owing to the expense of maintaining travelling home teachers, the limited amount of money available, and the widespread territory that had to be covered, it was found impossible to meet the demands for instruction that were constantly arising. Hence it was that in 1919, when the Canadian National Institute for the

Blind organized the Maritime Division of the Institute, it was agreed to have the income of the fund administered by the Board of Managers of the Maritime Division of the Canadian National Institute for the Blind. By this arrangement at least three home teachers of the blind may be kept constantly at work.

Although it is thought that the Montreal Association for the Blind may have provided occasional instruction in some homes in the vicinity of Montreal, Quebec did not have a formal home teaching program until the CNIB began to organize services in the province in 1930.

In Manitoba, toward the end of the First World War, the partially sighted Miss Alice Smith placed an ad in the newspaper offering to teach any blind person to read and write braille, free of charge. "Through this advertisement," Smith wrote, "I heard of four persons — a doctor, a young girl with partial sight, a blind girl, and a blind man." She gave these four instruction, and later, after the CNIB was formed in 1918, she became the first member of the home teaching staff of the organization. She also organized a social club called Lux in Tenebris ("Light in Darkness") for her blind pupils.

Newfoundland's development followed a different course. First a British protectorate, then an independent territory with its own government, it did not join Confederation until 1949. To its north across the Strait of Belle Isle lies Labrador. Although part of Newfoundland, Labrador is similar in demographics to the three other northern territories mentioned earlier. The reality is that it has proved very expensive to serve blind people who live in isolated, barely accessible communities.

Not surprisingly, the result is that in all four territories, despite the CNIB's best efforts, blind adults and youth continue to be disenfranchised.

As for the aboriginal populations of the far north, although reference is often made to their having an oral culture, they do in fact have written languages, but these cannot be written or read in braille, as braille codes have not been created for them.

By contrast, life as a blind person in central Canada — Ontario and Quebec — was much easier, and especially so if you happened to live in a larger city.

At Pearson Hall, the war-blinded veterans had been given instruction in braille, typing, crafts (including shoe repair), and massage therapy skills.

They were also given rehabilitation training, which helped them relearn how to do the simple things they had taken for granted when they were sighted, such as personal grooming, household tasks, shopping, and cooking. They also received orientation and mobility training, so they could get about safely and independently — not an easy task using a bamboo cane (it was not until much later that the white cane came into use).

CLASSES BEGIN

The first home teaching sponsored by the CNIB took place in Toronto, Hamilton, and Ingersoll. Charles Holmes, the CNIB director, had found three young blind women and engaged them to go into homes to teach blind people reading and simple crafts. Julia Dickson worked in Toronto, Emma Rooke visited homes in Hamilton, and Enid Loop taught in Ingersoll. The CNIB's first annual report records the instruction of 116 pupils over a period of 14 months.

In the spring of 1920, a training class for home teachers was organized in Toronto. Holmes had persuaded Julia Ward, a home teacher in Boston, to take on the job of chief instructor. Six prospective teachers enrolled in the program: the three teachers named above, who were already at work in the field, and three newcomers, Elizabeth Rusk, Nora Heaphy, and Eleanor Wooldridge. Classes were held in third floor rooms at 38 Adelaide Street West, next to the Blind Women's Industrial Workshop.

The curriculum consisted of braille reading, Moon type, groove card writing, typewriting, the making of reed baskets, willow baskets, and raffia mats, chair caning, netting (fish and tennis), hand sewing, machine sewing, knitting, and crocheting. Students also received instruction in heredity, biology, and psychology.

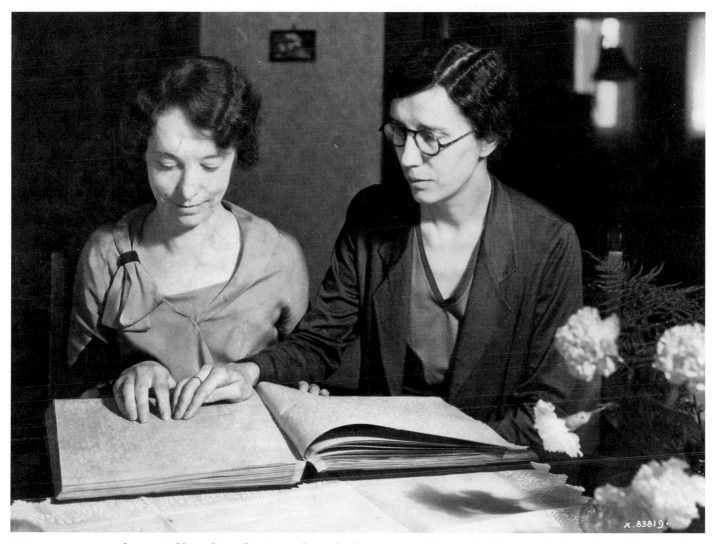

Home teacher Elizabeth Rusk, right, teaches Edna Sharpe to read braille, 1934.

The course lasted just over four months, until July 9, and Elizabeth Rusk went immediately to work in Toronto, taking over from Julia Dickson, who, for rea- sons unknown, was obliged to give up home teaching at that time.

The following year, Alice Smith, now Mrs. Richardson, was brought in from the Western division to

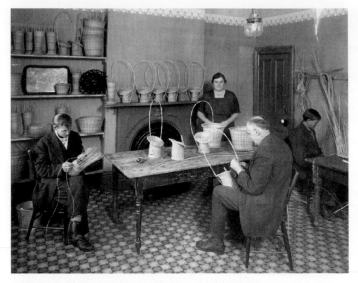

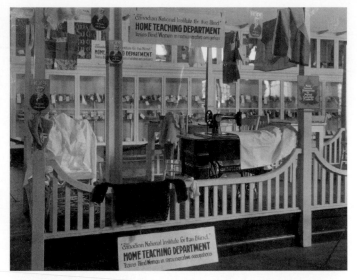

Mrs. Alwell instructs blind men in basketry in a CNIB work-room at 119 Spadina Avenue in Toronto, 1922.

A CNIB home teaching depart-ment exhibit at the Canadian National Exhibition in Toronto, 1922.

teach the second class of fourteen teachers in training — two from Nova Scotia, six from Ontario, three from Saskatchewan, one from Alberta, and two from British Columbia.

Richardson was later to remark that she knew so little about basketry she had to take lessons at night so she could stay one step ahead of her students.

It's important to note that in the 1920s, baskets and reed (or willow) furniture were fashionable, and the hope was that if a blind person could become proficient in

this type of work, he might be able to earn an income, or even a living, from it.

Besides skills and crafts, the home teachers also helped their students with the physical and psychological adjustment to the loss of sight.

The CNIB teachers were all women, and all were blind or severely visually impaired; they eventually performed their duties with assistance from sighted guides who also acted as drivers. In the United States, the occupation of home teaching was open to men and women alike, whereas in Great Britain, most of the home teachers were sighted women.

In her Master of Social Work thesis of 1948, CNIB home teacher and later National Director of Welfare Services and Home Teaching Louise Cowan describes the attributes and qualifications a home teacher of the blind should have:

> She must herself have made a comfortable adjustment to blindness — free from self-pity and from morbid concern for other blind. She should possess sound general intelligence, average academic rating, better than average initiative and imagination … She must determine what is the right psychological approach, what hobbies or regular tasks are best suited to the particular individual. The home teacher has a special job to do and for the most part she has to do it alone.

> She should be carefully groomed because she represents to many the ultimate accomplishment of intelligent blind women.

Cowan also made special mention of the fact that home teaching was not just for adults. Preschool children benefited from home teaching, too, although Cowan recommended that a social worker be brought in to work with the parents, leaving the home teacher free to focus on the child: "Her work with the child would also demonstrate to the parents the methods used in working with a blind person and something of the achievement of the blind adult."

In her thesis, Cowan describes the case of Roget, a little blind boy, using information supplied by Ms. S. Miller, a home teacher in Windsor, Ontario:

> Roget, who was born blind, was first visited by the home teacher when he was six or seven years old. The mother, who had two other small children to care for,

knew nothing about blindness and did not know how to begin training her little boy. The home teacher visited her several times before convincing her that Roget could be taught to walk, feed himself and go about the house by himself as other children did. She let Roget sit in a rocking chair for part of the day until she found time to put his clothes on. He had an appetite like a man and was becoming quite fat and clumsy. He was not allowed to go anywhere outside or inside the house by himself.

After a period of about seven weeks, with three to four visits each week, the home teacher was able to have Roget find his way through the house, walk around the block, do a bit of marching, name all the common objects with which he came in contact, and sing a few little songs.

When I look back and see how much Roget did in this short time I am amazed, and the father, mother and two small sisters now realize that Roget should in a short time be able to live a normal life with them.

In the 1940s, veterans blinded in the combat theatres of the Second World War were being sent home in higher numbers than during the 1914–1918 conflict. By then, however, the CNIB was in a position to offer training independently of St Dunstan's or any other facility. Thanks to the generosity of Lady Virginia Kemp, who had been a dedicated volunteer and benefactor from the institute's inception, the CNIB had acquired a beautiful house on Admiral Road in central Toronto, which it named Baker Hall. It was here that blind servicemen went to receive rehabilitation training. Elizabeth Rusk, who had been in the first class of 1920, was one of their teachers.

Baker Hall, which had been purchased outright for the CNIB and placed in a trust, was later transferred to the CNIB when the veterans' rehabilitation programs were completed. After the war, civilians were trained there until 1956, when the BakerWood complex was opened at 1929 Bayview Avenue in Toronto.

PROFESSIONAL STANDARDS

By the 1930s, the CNIB had been operating a home teaching program for well over ten years. Managing director Colonel E.A. Baker acknowledged the sterling work being done by the home teachers but also noted that the service was inconsistent: some districts had no home teaching at all, and in others the service provided was inadequate.

To improve the quality of the work being done in the field, and to attract the kind of intelligent, educated, and responsible women the CNIB wanted for its home teaching program, the organization decided to formalize its home teaching program, beginning with a survey to establish needs and criteria.

In 1938, representatives from Canadian and American agencies for the blind met in New York to discuss uniform and improved standards for home teaching. Out of this conference came a comprehensive list of academic requirements that a prospective home teacher of the blind would need to meet to qualify for a Class I certificate. Requirements for a Class II certificate were also set out.

Because of the intervening Second World War, the CNIB was not able to begin providing all the training necessary for certification until the summer of 1945.

The members of the 1947 class not only completed the academic and practical requirements of their program but also went on to form an association for all Canadian home teachers, called the Canadian Association of Rehabilitation Teachers (CART), with a members' publication, called *Our Rendezvous*. CART was accepted as an internal association by the CNIB senior management and was provided with funding and regular conferences.

In 1951, the CNIB recruited Dr. S.A. Saunders to establish a formal national training program, which was expanded beyond the training of home teachers to include vocational training and

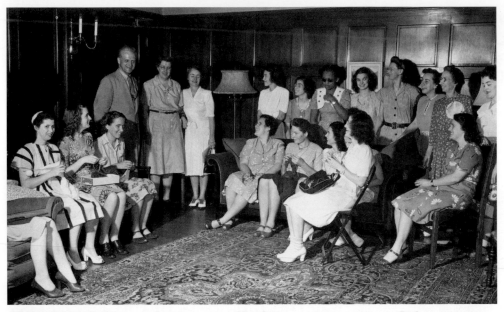

Edwin Baker shares a light moment with members of the CNIB home teachers training class, 1947.

trained specialists were employed by school boards and other blindness organizations, the decision was taken to phase out both in-house training of specialists and the certification requirements.

The CNIB continued to operate its training program for home teachers, and to certify them, until the late 1980s, when the work was taken over by an Ontario college.

courses in administration for field personnel and middle management. Also in 1951, the home teaching program accepted men for the first time, when Elwood Greenfield of Saskatchewan and Oscar Amyotte of Ontario became the first male home teachers.

The issue of certification for "agency-trained" rehabilitation specialists versus the American university-based training model remained contentious and controversial for at least fifty years. For complex reasons, not least of which were issues of potential liability when CNIB-

Mohawk College, located in Brantford, Ontario, offers two specialized programs that train instructors to work with blind and visually impaired clients of all ages and with a variety of physical or learning disabilities. These programs, Instructor for Blind & Visually Impaired — Orientation and Mobility and Instructor for Blind & Visually Impaired — Rehabilitation, are the only full-time English-language programs of their kind in Canada. In

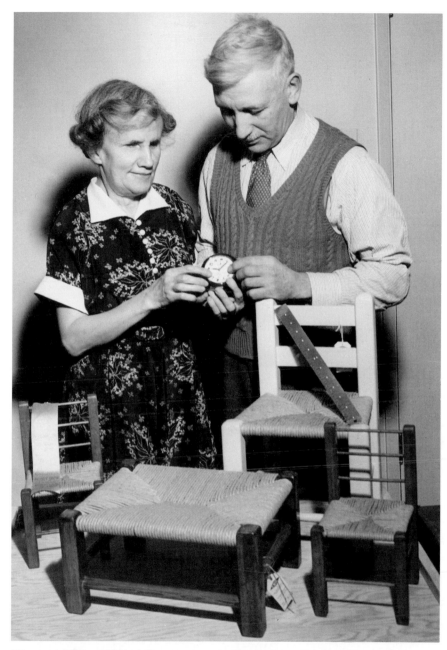

Dorothy Stark was a home teacher in the B.C-Yukon division from about 1930 to the late 1950s.

Quebec, similar French-language training programs have been offered.

No amount of praise or admiration can adequately acknowledge the contribution and pioneering spirit of these early home teachers of the blind. They were far ahead of their time, long before community-based rehabilitation was ever thought of.

The patience, caring, and success rate of these teachers, who were mostly young and mostly women, is beyond measure. They overcame all kinds of logistical problems to reach their students, bringing with them hope and help.

Over the years, the elements of rehabilitation were expanded and adjusted as social conditions evolved. What never varied, however, is instruction in fundamental life skills. Rehabilitation teachers and instructors have always been central to CNIB programs.

CHAPTER 7
Working Toward Gainful Employment

For most adults, occupational status — the work we do — helps define who we are. Well paid, meaningful work that allows us to use our skills, gifts, and abilities and that brings financial security and stability to our lives is the key to achieving self-realization and fulfillment.

But for many Canadian working-age adults who are blind or visually impaired, the opportunity to compete for jobs and obtain gainful, competitive employment was a long time coming — and

still, the employment rate for blind and visually impaired Canadians remains lower than for the general population.

In the 1980s and 1990s, governments at the provincial and federal levels introduced public policies, legislation, and regulatory provisions that mandated employment accessibility for Canadians with disabilities. The private sector then moved gradually, and sometimes reluctantly, to open up hundreds of different positions, which, until then, would have been considered off limits to someone who was blind or visually impaired. Opportunities on factory floors and at boardroom tables opened up.

This was in sharp contrast to the way it had been a century earlier.

By the mid-nineteenth century in Europe, blind men were obtaining employment independently, mostly as musicians or in cottage industry craft production. Organized industrial workshops for the blind became common by the end of the nineteenth century in many parts of the world, including Canada. A few talented blind men, such as Louis Braille, had also managed to find employment in the professions, for example teaching in the schools for the blind. An accomplished organist, Braille taught music at the prestigious Institut National des Jeunes Aveugles in Paris. Some blind people who had acquired certain skills became piano tuners, masseurs, farmers, or street vendors — jobs that over time grew to be stereotypes analogous to basket weaving.

But for most blind people the grim reality was that on leaving a school for the blind, either as a graduate or upon having reached the age of majority, there was not much they could do except return to their home communities with few prospects of obtaining rewarding, enjoyable work that would make them financially independent. They would be forced to rely on their families to support them for all the years to come.

It was within this bleak context that private associations set out to create employment opportunities for people who were blind or visually impaired.

By about 1915, broom making workshops offering employment to blind men had opened, and within a decade, shops in Halifax, Ottawa, Toronto, Montreal, Vancouver, and Winnipeg were in full operation. Exactly why the manufacture of brooms and brushes, which involves sharp, spinning blades, was considered suitable work for blind men isn't known.

Other products, like mattresses, were manufactured by men working in sheltered workshops. Eventually, blind men were producing such diverse goods as fire starters in Vancouver and claim stakes in Calgary, as well as packaging commercial products, from soap to nuts, on a piece basis.

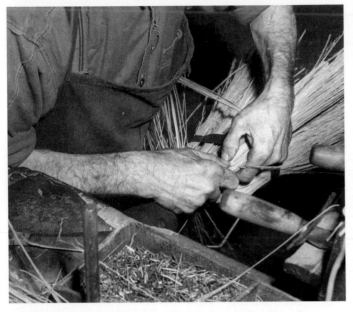

In the early days of the twentieth century, broom making was considered a suitable job for blind men.

Several of these shops predated the CNIB's founding in 1918, but realizing the importance of such programs, the CNIB management moved to acquire them. In Winnipeg, Vancouver, and several Ontario cities, the CNIB established shops early on. Other shops, such as those in Newfoundland and Quebec, would not become part of the CNIB's operations for another ten years or so.

Workshops for blind women were few and far between.

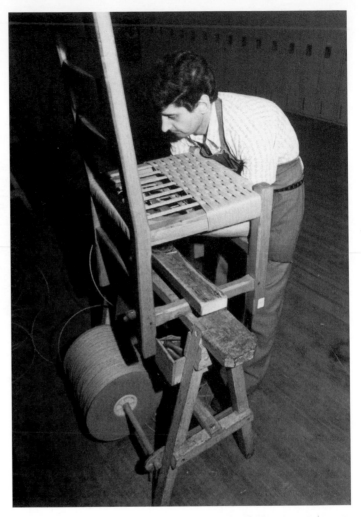

Chair caning was a highly prized skill.

There was one in Toronto, however, and the women who worked there made an outstanding contribution to the war effort, as this excerpt from the July 1940 issue of the *National News of the Blind* shows.

The employees of the apron and dress factory of The Canadian National Institute for the Blind in Toronto have undertaken to look after one war guest. There are, at the present time, forty-one blind girls and women employed in this plant and they have, in conjunction with the sighted girls who work with them, made

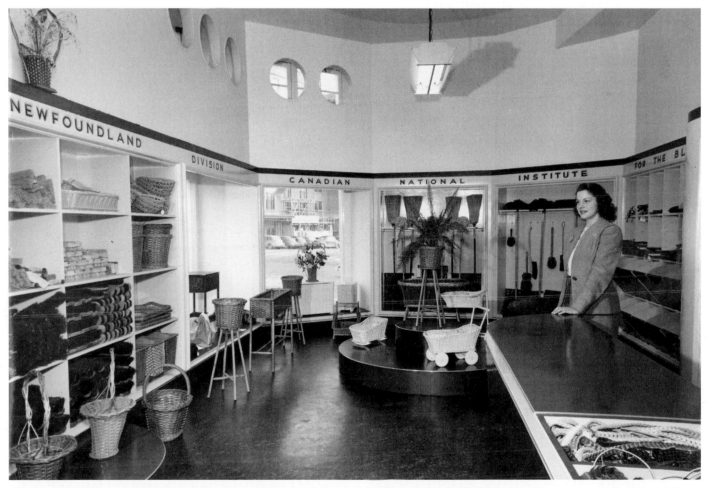

The spacious Blindcraft shop of St. John's, Newfoundland, 1948. All goods, including brooms, brushes, and baskets, would have been made by blind people.

arrangements to provide the necessary funds for the maintenance of one of the children now coming to Canada from England …

At the start of the war this same group of girls, working in their spare time, made hundreds of pyjamas for the use of children evacuated from British cities. Since then they have given freely of their services, working in conjunction with the Canadian Red Cross and the Daughters of the Empire. Recently they made and gave to the Red Cross eighty-six girls' dresses for the English children arriving in Canada.

A garment factory employing blind women also flourished in Winnipeg for many years until the mid-1970s.

Most of these shops struggled to make a profit, as blind workers manufactured the brooms and then were expected to go door to door to sell them. Often, failure to meet sales targets meant that the suppliers of raw materials could not be paid. In Halifax, that scenario forced the shop to close. In other cases, the CNIB's national office had to rob Peter to pay Paul — juggling funds from one part of the country to another to balance out the viability of these operations.

Managing the finances of the broom shops was no doubt a daunting challenge for a young organization that needed ever increasing sources of funds to meet a growing appetite for training, capital acquisitions, and employment programs.

In 1923, thirty-year-old Edwin Baker was far wiser and more visionary than his years would suggest. From his broad network of contacts in Europe and the United States, from his two years in Ottawa advising the federal government on rehabilitation of the war-blinded, and most of all from his own experience, he was aware of the importance of employment for blind people.

By 1925 he had determined that employment opportunities for both civilian and war-blinded men had to be broadened. As for women, society had few expectations of them or opportunities for them beyond home, church, and perhaps a little genteel charity work, and how well they did in life was tied to marriage, not education and employment. Blind women in those days were marginalized and would remain so for generations. Helen Keller, the deaf-blind American advocate for the rights of blind people, was a striking exception.

Employment of the blind followed two streams: sheltered employment within the CNIB or gradually expanding opportunities to be found in society at large.

Through a careful, selective process the CNIB identified blind men and women who were considered suitable for advancement and offered extensive training programs for rehabilitation workers, administrators, and executives, something the organization would continue to do over the next eighty years.

People thought unsuitable, or those who fell outside the CNIB's corporate mould for whatever reason, however, had little hope of inclusion on this career path.

By 1930, a training and employment placement program was well-established at the national office in Toronto. As the CNIB's geographic divisions evolved, they developed employment placement programs to complement the programs offered by the national office.

Together, they pioneered training programs in new fields. For example, it is thought that blind darkroom technicians were first trained at the Royal Victoria Hospital in Montreal, opening up job opportunities nationwide at competitive salaries in this field.

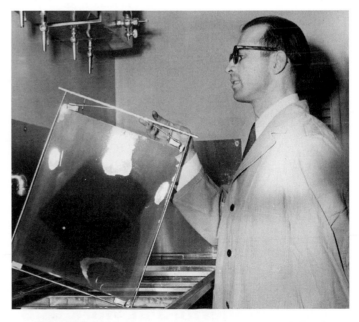

A blind man working as a highly skilled film developer, Royal Victoria Hospital, Montreal.

Over many years, blind Canadians received professional training at the RNIB in London. University-based training in Canada for blind physiotherapists was only marginally successful.

In the early days of the twentieth century, when secretaries and typists produced letters and other documents, dicta typing was considered suitable work for blind people, usually women. In dicta typing, someone would dictate a letter or report into a recording

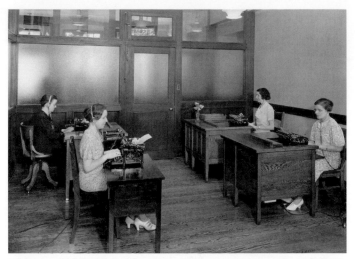

The CNIB dictaphone pool, 186 Beverley Street, Toronto.

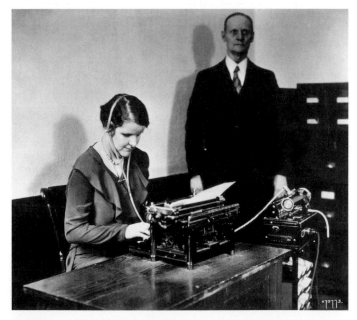

Lillian Hungerford at work as a dictaphone typist in the Howard Smith Paper Mills in Montreal, 1931.

machine, and the dicta typist, listening to the recorded voice through earphones, would type the required document. The CNIB offered a dicta typing training program, and in fact, Baker's first job when he returned to Canada as a war-blinded veteran was as a dicta typist with the Ontario Hydro Electric Power Commission.

Once qualified, blind dicta typists were sought-after in hospitals and medical clinics, and this proved to be a worthwhile career for generations of blind women. For many years, dating back to at least 1920, letters sent from the CNIB often carried the following message at the bottom: "This letter was dictated to the Dictaphone and transcribed by a blind typist."

The message usually had a powerful impact on sighted recipients.

Although the CNIB had only limited success placing blind people in jobs in the 1920s because of resistance from employers, in 1932 it placed its first dicta typist in a job in London.

CLUNK AND WILLIAMSON

The annual conventions of the American Association of Workers for the Blind eventually included delegates from Canada, and Baker and subsequent CNIB leaders attended regularly. It is likely from this network that Joe F. Clunk came to the attention of the CNIB senior management. Clunk, a blind lawyer from the United States, was hired by the CNIB in 1928 to develop an employment placement program. Both Clunk and Baker had an uncanny gift for identifying talent and leadership in others.

Clunk's approach to job searching was straightforward and effective. He made cold calls on industry at a senior level and asked for

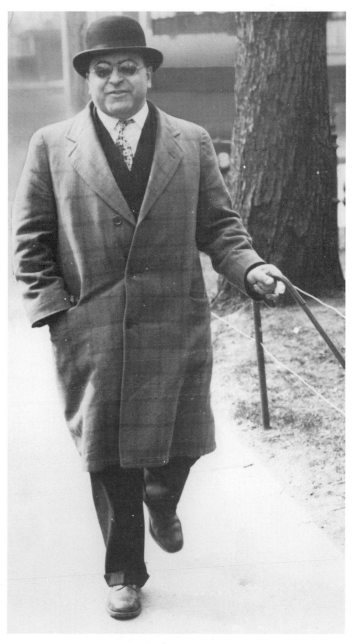

A jaunty Joe Clunk, supervisor of industrial placements and aftercare for Toronto.

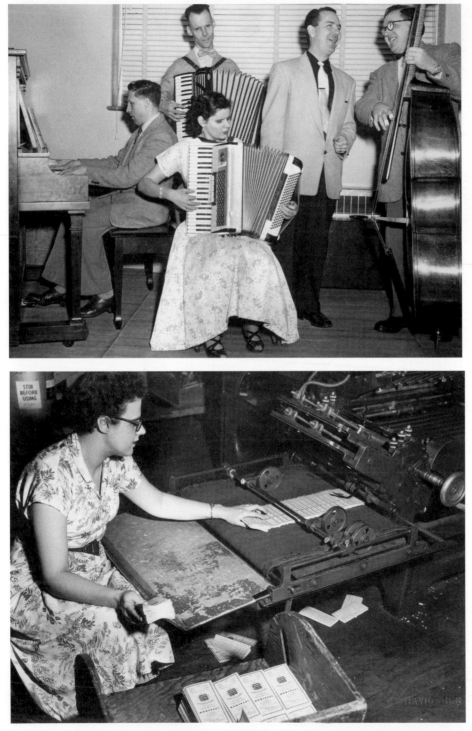

an opportunity to demonstrate on the assembly line or factory floor how a blind person could handle a job safely and on a par with a sighted worker. Once Clunk had proved that a blind person could do the job, the door was open for a blind person to be trained to do that job. This opened interesting jobs in industries such as steel, automotive assembly, and

TOP: Blind musicians in 1957. The piano player, Herb Essenberg, is the little boy in the front row in the photo of the school percussion band in Chapter 1.

BOTTOM: A blind woman working in the printing industry at a counting and bundling machine in the 1950s.

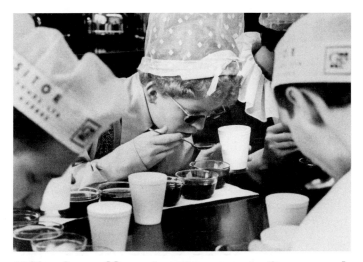

Blind coffee tasters at General Foods, 1971.

manufacturing that had previously been thought off limits.

The diversity of jobs blind people began to undertake was amazing.

One man, with very limited vision, was employed by a Toronto ice company. As trainloads of bacon rolled east to Halifax for export during the Second World War, this man's job was to pitch bags of ice into open railroad cars to refrigerate the meat.

Clunk has been described as outgoing, even aggressive, and his nature was at times out of step with the more conservative culture of the CNIB. Clunk travelled the country by himself in search of new openings.

It was on such a trip to Vancouver that he met Lindsay Williamson. Born into a Saskatchewan ranching family, Williamson moved with his parents to the Arrow Lakes area near Nelson, British Columbia, as a young boy. His vision deteriorated rapidly, and by the age of eighteen he was completely blind. Both his parents having died within a year in 1925, Williamson found market gardening too difficult and turned to producing wooden water pipe. Seven-foot-by-five-inch jack pine logs were hollowed out and attached into lengths and sold for domestic use and irrigation.

Three years later, he was hired to work in the CNIB original broom shop in Vancouver's False Creek. A year later, a new building on Broadway combining shops and offices was opened, and Williamson was asked to manage the workshop program, including product development and sales. It was here that Clunk was intro-duced to Williamson, and soon after, in 1929, Williamson was per-suaded to move to Toronto.

Williamson says he began his

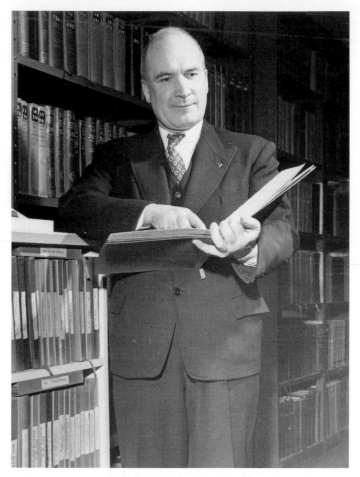

Lindsay Williamson, national director of employment services, 1947.

Clunk and Williamson on board, who could have predicted the long-range outcomes of their determination, hard work, and conviction that blind workers were entitled to economic independence and financial security?

They, with additional staff recruited from the provinces, in the height of the Depression and against nearly insurmountable odds, changed the face of work for the blind in Canada forever.

This integration into the workplace, in many respects, led the industrialized world and broke the stereotypical mould that blind people qualified for only a narrow range of occupations.

In Toronto, Williamson was given a portfolio of photos showing blind workers who had been successfully placed, and with this under his arm, he was sent into industry to show the photos to potential employers as examples of what could be done. Only a person with inner strength and initiative could have accepted the challenge as the Great Depression of the 1930s was settling over the Canadian landscape. Later in his career, in a charmingly folksy way, Williamson recounted an

on-the-job training as the CNIB's second placement officer on his first train trip to Toronto, when they stopped off in Regina and Winnipeg to explore job opportunities. As the Vancouver train steamed into Union Station in Toronto in 1930 with assignment that he had been given in 1931:

The second time I was given a real job to do. There was a [blind] chap living up in the Kirkland Lake district, Northern Ontario, up in the mining country, and he wanted a job. He couldn't be moved down, he was married and tied up there pretty well and it was important that he get something to do.

So Mr. Clunk said to me, "How would you like to go up to Kirkland Lake and find this chap a job up there? There must be something he can do in some of those mines and if you can't find him a job in the mine, maybe you can find room for a little kiosk or stand somewhere on a busy corner and we could place him selling cigarettes and candy bars."

I said I would do the best I could because during our training period that was my job as well — securing stands and kiosks and placing them and setting people up in their own businesses. I had quite a catalogue of jobs to attend to.

So the wife packed my little grip for me and I got my ticket and I was off to Kirkland Lake. And Joe Clunk told me not to come back until I had got this chap sorted out with a job.

[We couldn't get him a job in the mine], and there weren't any industries in the town, it was all mines, so I said I'll try something else. I'd called on this blind chap and he was rather a nice chap and he struck me as a person who would be much better suited to operating a small business, so I said well, the town was big enough to support a stand of this sort.

So I looked around

the town, as a blind man looks, asking questions and using his cane and so they mentioned to me just on the main corner was the United Church so I thought well, this looks like a good spot, and I listened to the traffic and asked a lot of questions and thought he might sell a lot of things. So we got the approval, and hunted up carpenters and supervised the building of the kiosk. And the chap said he'd like that much better than working up at the mine, so I said all right, that's your job.

By now I'd been away a month and my wife was getting worried and Colonel Baker was getting worried.

But the boy worked there for quite a long time, and then we placed another blind person in the same stand, so that was another job for another blind person.

But I'm telling you, it was no easy job for a totally blind person to travel alone in territory he doesn't know a thing about, miles from anywhere. Now going up to Kirkland Lake, in those days the train didn't run into Kirkland Lake but only went to Swastika, a little town about 10 miles out of Kirkland Lake. And the train that I traveled on got into Swastika about 1 a.m.

And my trip was in the dead of winter and there was a lot of snow and no station, and the conductor told me there was nothing there, only an old boxcar which acts as a station.

So I hopped off the train and away she went. I landed in two feet of snow, and I got my little cane walloping around there, and I'd step off the track a bit and pretty soon I came to what felt like a little sidewalk.

So I ran my cane and felt the door and opened it and stepped in. A fellow said, "Hey, where you going?" And he said you can't get to Kirkland Lake until ten in the morning. So I said well, I got to stay. You've got a bench here, haven't you? He said yeah, and I said what about you? And he said I got to stay here and keep the fire going. So I said, well, I'll sleep on the bench.

But when I hopped off that train and stood in one place until the train was out of hearing distance there must have been about forty-six wolves that started to howl all at once, and there's me in two feet of snow, not knowing where I was. My hair was standing straight up even though I had a heavy cap on. It was all pioneer work in those days and it wasn't easy but it was work that I loved.

In 1935, after working for the CNIB for seven years, Clunk returned to the United States, leaving the employment program well-established in Toronto and placement officers recruited in several divisions. The dedicated Williamson worked for thirty-five years building the employment department until his retirement in 1963.

STANDS AND CANTEENS

In 1928, blind men began operating street units or stands located in office building lobbies from which they sold various goods such as tobacco, chocolate bars, newspapers, and sometimes handicraft items produced by blind people. Initially, these were operator-owned with minimal standards for accounting and hygiene, but they did change the image of a blind beggar on the street to an entrepreneur with high visibility.

Started in Toronto, the network of stands spread to other cities once Baker had broken down the federal government's initial reluctance to allow blind veterans to operate stands in government buildings. Eventually, the CNIB had

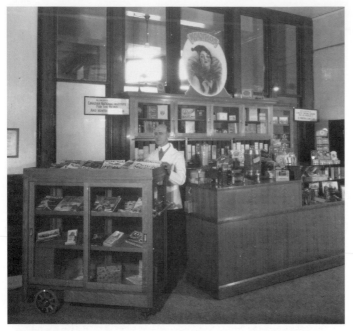

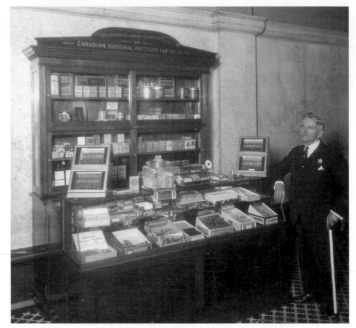

A blind man operates a stand selling tobacco and sweets at the Montreal General Hospital, 1931.

This stand did a good business at the courthouse in Vancouver, British Columbia, 1932.

first refusal in most federal public buildings in every province, and many blind men spent their entire working lives operating a stand.

The resourceful Clunk is also credited with helping blind people establish and operate cafeterias and canteens in industrial or commercial establishments. In 1929, aware that it was almost impossible to obtain factory jobs for blind men because there were thousands of skilled workers competing for jobs, Clunk decided that there was no reason why, given the right training and support, blind men should not operate a little counter over which they could dispense coffee, sandwiches, and easily prepared snacks. From this small beginning a full-fledged cafeteria system developed, and by 1940, one hundred blind men and women across Canada were operating canteens and cafeterias under the auspices of the CNIB.

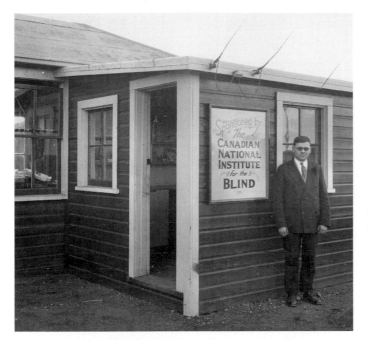

Paul Chudek operates a stand constructed for him by Canadian Pacific Railway workers in Calgary, Alberta.

In 1934, recruited by Clunk, Doug Strong joined the CNIB. A graduate engineer, Strong was blinded when the car in which he was a passenger struck a bridge abutment. Amazingly, ten years later, in 1942, medical treatment successfully restored almost all of his vision.

Following on-the-job training, Strong was put in charge of the stand program, and he developed operating and accounting standards

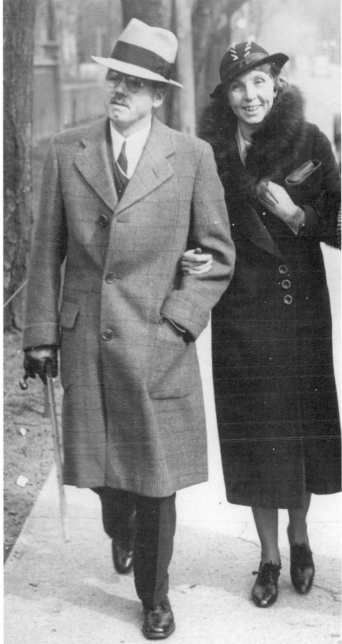

Doug Strong with his sister Florence.

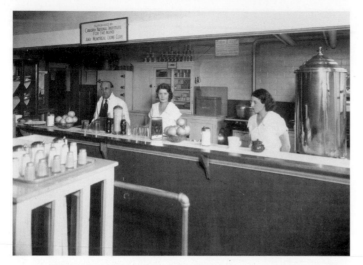

A CaterPlan operation at Dawes Brewery in Montreal, 1932.

for the canteens. By now, the program had moved from the street corner and building lobbies and had gradually expanded into full-size food operations and cafeterias.

CaterPlan, as it became known, was a CNIB program designed to employ as many blind people as possible, although sighted workers were hired to perform jobs for which sight was thought to be essential, such as food handling and some senior management positions.

The outbreak of the Second World War brought new opportunities for catering at large plants producing goods needed for the war effort. Strong had been to the United States to see how this kind of operation was run, and the Canadian program was modelled on the U.S. experience. Throughout the war, good contacts and shrewd, leveraged negotiations ensured the CNIB had access to highly prized items such as cigarettes, sugar, candy bars, and gasoline, which were in short supply elsewhere because of strict rationing.

During the course of Strong's thirty-four years with the CNIB, cafeteria sales grew by leaps and bounds. In 1934, gross sales totalled $500,000; by 1968, the year Strong retired, annual sales had reached $24 million. By 1980, the combined annual cash flow of CaterPlan and the workshops exceeded $44 million.

In 1968, CNIB operated at some 550 locations in every part of Canada, including the military installation in Churchill, Manitoba. There were 750 blind people working in 275 canteens and 2,100 sighted employees serving mostly in cafeterias in industrial plants such as Stelco in Hamilton, at Hydro Quebec, in federal buildings, and in the Canadian Broadcasting Corporation. The largest operations by far were in Ontario and Quebec.

By the late 1960s, CaterPlan was renowned as one of the largest industrial cafeteria operations in Canada. Success knew few boundaries. Commercial kitchens at BakerWood, with a fleet of delivery trucks, supplied hot meals and baked goods to local businesses. On occasion, long-distance delivery was even undertaken. In the summer of 1967, CaterPlan staff in Toronto were asked to provide refreshments for the opening of the National Gallery in Ottawa, an important centennial event to be attended by Prime Minister Lester B. Pearson and twelve hundred other guests.

The food was prepared in the BakerWood kitchen — one hundred dozen stuffed finger rolls, five thousand sandwiches, and thousands of petit fours, cookies, and other treats — and then trucked four hundred kilometres to Ottawa in time for the event. Silverware, punch bowls, and non-perishable foods had been delivered the day before. To further illustrate the CNIB's reach in the catering industry, it was contracted to redesign the kitchens of Rideau Hall, the

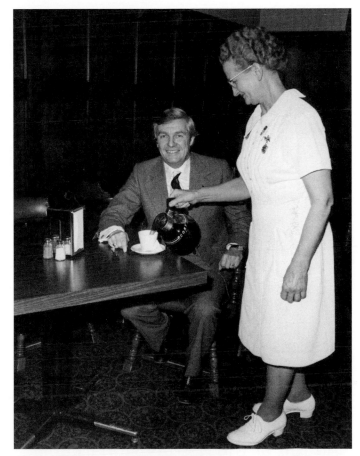

The Honourable Peter Lougheed, premier of Alberta, being served coffee by Vera Shepherd, manager of the CaterPlan Legislative Cafeteria, 1976.

Governor General's official residence in Ottawa.

An early signal of CaterPlan's demise may well have been a costly but failed experiment to open a commercial restaurant, the

Witness Box, in Toronto. This fully licensed establishment, which opened amid high hopes on University Avenue across from the courthouse and close to law offices and Osgoode Hall in the spring of 1972, was designed to provide revenue for rehabilitation programs as well as employment for blind people.

By the year 2000, with the exception of the four Atlantic provinces, CaterPlan had been either sold to private entrepreneurs or simply phased out. Also by then, industrial and occupational workshops located in most provinces had been closed.

Later chapters are needed to unravel the internal and external factors that account for the rise and fall of these truly remarkable programs in essentially less than sixty years.

Beyond question, though, for half a century the catering program was a fertile recruiting ground for CNIB management at all levels. Field men, provincial directors, and rehab personnel all started their CNIB careers in the program, some as students. The five men who succeeded Baker as president and CEO of the CNIB

started in the canteens: Art Magill, Ross Purse, Robert Mercer, Euclid Herie, and Jim Sanders.

For others, including Strong, employment in the stand program was part of training and rehabilitation as individuals were moved into administration and other duties within the CNIB.

Williamson and Strong, in their own fields and their own ways, left huge footprints on the landscape of employment of the blind.

BLIND WORKMAN'S COMPENSATION ACT

In 1931, "to provide special protection for employers of blind workers and to encourage the employment of blind in general industrial occupations," the Ontario government passed the Blind Workman's Compensation Act. The real purpose of the act, however, as explained within it, was to "encourage the employment of blind workmen by relieving employers of the apprehension they might otherwise be under of employing blind workmen and thereby increasing the possibility of accident and compensation."

The bill provided for compensation to blind workmen for injuries sustained and industrial diseases contracted in the course of their employment. Under its terms, the CNIB was charged with "proper industrial placement of the blind," which meant that the CNIB "shall have exclusive jurisdiction as to the nature of the work a blind workman shall do and as to the proper placement of such a workman." For some blind workers, this clause no doubt limited personal choice. An employer giving employment to a blind workman without the consent or approval of the institute, or changing the nature of the blind employee's work, would not be protected by the act.

An important dimension related to the employment of blind workers was gaining the cooperation and acceptance of unions within collective bargaining agreements. In some cases, shop unions agreed to exempt a blind worker from bumping provisions of a collective agreement to protect the designated job. Here, too, the blind worker may have been locked into one job, limiting or excluding mobility sideways or

vertically. But despite the limitations, it was solid employment and economic security unprecedented in history.

Without doubt, this act created a comfort level for employers, at the same time limiting their potential financial liability. With the emergence of other generic legislation dealing with human rights and employment standards, opportunities and jobs in industry were opened up for blind workers.

Workman's Compensation Boards in other provinces supported similar legislation, some of which remained in force until the 1980s. Gradually, however, as the social climate changed, each act was repealed as industry accepted that such protective measures were no longer necessary or appropriate. Besides levelling the playing field for blind and sighted workers, the repeals also gave blind workers, male or female, the chance to obtain employment independently without the knowledge and consent of the CNIB.

Community-based training and education programs for blind adults appeared in the 1960s. Shifting public attitudes and growing awareness, spawned by government initiatives and funding known as "affirmative action," became an adjunct to the CNIB's own programs.

In the late 1960s, when computer programming was in its infancy, the University of Manitoba offered customized training for blind people that launched many into successful careers. Many of the graduates, who would not even have qualified for university admission in the normal way, were sought-after by government and private sector employers. Others pursued this career through regular computer science courses.

One person who deserves credit for his role in helping blind people take their place in the workforce is blind scientist James Swail, who invented or adapted more than thirty devices that help blind people at work.

Blinded at the age of four in an automobile accident, Swail had to push his way through barriers while still in high school. As a high school student he was not allowed to take laboratory work in chemistry, so he built his own lab at home. He was accepted into McGill University and graduated with a B.Sc.

He began his career with the National Research Council of Canada in Ottawa in 1947, and over the years he designed more than thirty aids for blind people that had practical workplace applications. His devices included an electronic thermometer with a raised scale for reading by touch and an audible tone to indicate fluid levels, which made it possible for a blind person to monitor the temperatures of developing solutions in a photographic darkroom. He used the same principle to adapt electronic meters, which opened up opportunities for blind people in broadcast engineering, motor repair, and assembly-line inspections in electronics industries. In the days before computers he also created a braille slide rule, a carpenter's level, and an audio indicator for tape recorders. He was also instrumental in developing a computer punch card system for blind programmers, in the pioneering days of computer technology. Swail was awarded the Order of Canada.

In the absence of a proactive employment training program for the blind within the government sector, the playing field largely remained with the CNIB until the 1980s. The introduction of the Canada Assistance Plan by the federal government in 1966 laid the groundwork for legislation and revenue sharing with the provinces that would change the social landscape for all Canadians, including those with disabilities. As an outgrowth of this federal policy, a contractual agreement between the provinces and the federal government on public sector funding for employment and vocational training of the disabled took root.

The Vocational Rehabilitation of Disabled Persons Act (VRDP) provided what became known as "fifty-cent dollars." Under this scheme, the federal government matched every fifty cents spent by the provinces on vocational rehabilitation.

The program worked very well despite protracted negotiations almost every year among authorities and end-user organizations. However, the catch was that the province had to pony up its fifty cents first in order to receive matching funds, which in some cases led to delays in launching new initiatives. Eventually, through negotiations, there were well-trained, qualified employment counsellors who understood the special needs of blind students and employees in each CNIB division for thirty years.

By contrast, counsellors at the Canada Manpower Centres of the day were too ill-prepared and ill-trained to be of significant support. In theory, although every Canadian working age adult had a right to all the support and information a Manpower Centre could provide, the reality was that if you were blind or visually impaired, the CNIB was your only real service provider.

CHAPTER 8
The Seeds of Empowerment

William (Willy) Johnson attended a school for the blind in England and was trained as a piano tuner. In 1910, his family settled in Winnipeg, and in 1917 he joined the Winnipeg Piano Company as a tuner where he worked until 1925, when he decided to go into business for himself. Nearly sixty years later, Johnson was still tuning, repairing, and selling pianos throughout Manitoba. He also served on the CNIB's Manitoba division board for more than fifty-five years.

If you had met Willy Johnson, even in his later years, you would have noticed that he had a charmingly feisty and talkative manner. Although small in stature, he was large in every aspect of advocacy, legislation, and services to do with blindness.

"This is the blind calling," he would say in his best British accent as he introduced himself to a government minister, mayor, or any other official he telephoned to request a meeting or decision on an important issue.

Johnson also led the charge in the blindness consumer movement. The seeds of consumerism outside Toronto took root in the first decades of the twentieth century. Disabled First World War veterans had formed associations soon after their return to Canada, and the war-blinded were in the forefront of the movement.

For the civilian blind, however, formal organizations of blind adults were few and far between. Johnson would claim that he and three other blind people from England living in Winnipeg, including home teacher Alice Smith, chartered the first association of the blind when, in 1919, they formed the Lux in Tenebris Club. Shortly after, they petitioned the Manitoba government to form the Industrial Association of the Blind. Located in the Donalda Block of downtown Winnipeg, the association started a Dictaphone typist course and reported that they had placed two dicta typists with the Great-West Life Assurance Company by 1920.

In 1919, the CNIB sought to establish a division in Manitoba and recruited Samuel Robert Hussey, founder of the

Halifax Association of the Blind, to be the superintendent.

Johnson and his associates negotiated a precedent-setting agreement early on with the CNIB that their consumer association would no longer provide services but would take on a watchdog role and co-operate with the CNIB's board. In return for the CNIB's pro-

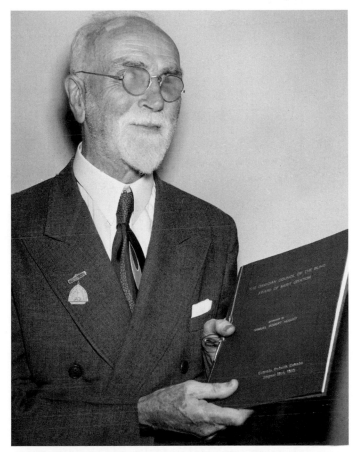

S.R. Hussey was given the first Award of Merit by the CCB.

viding financial support, the association agreed not to undertake competitive fundraising. This principle would come into play twenty-five years later when the Canadian Council of the Blind was formed.

This trade-off agreement was definitely not viewed as financial paternalism on the part of the CNIB but rather as a pragmatic accommodation or, in the parlance of the day, a gentlemen's agreement. It was a business deal.

Before long, to create better public awareness, the Lux In Tenebris Club changed its name to the Manitoba League of the Blind. The league then joined the Canadian Federation of the Blind, which had been formed by Philip Layton in 1926 in Montreal; it was at this point that a national consumer organization of the blind, complete with a federal charter, began to spread its reach across Canada.

Not surprisingly, the CFOB and the CNIB were soon locking horns as they competed to raise funds, win the hearts and minds of the public, and raise their profiles with governments.

To what extent this struggle became polarized on the fierce individuality and personalities of the CNIB's Baker and the CFOB's Layton is open to debate. However, the well-known rivalry and, at times, bitter public disagreements between the two groups continued into the late 1950s.

For its part, the CFOB established provincial chapters, sold a magazine called *Vision* on street corners to raise funds, established credible boards, and acquired property outside Quebec. When the CNIB organized in Saskatchewan, it acquired the CFOB's boards and residential facilities in Regina and Saskatoon.

A sorry footnote to the history of blindness in Canada is that both organizations had similar goals: they advocated for legislation, pensions, and jobs and wanted desperately to change public attitudes toward blind people. Both were led by high profile, competent, accomplished blind men, both employed blind men and women, and both had strong representation of blind people on their boards.

Why then, could they not find common ground and optimize their forces and resources?

The one time they did effectively join forces to lobby the

federal and provincial governments for pension legislation, the two organizations, along with others, eventually achieved a meeting of minds on strategy, amount of pension sought, and eligibility requirements.

It may be that the two organizations had difficulty working together because their leaders' egos could not accommodate such a partnership. It was more likely, however, that the real problem was the stiff competition for control of the precious few resources available.

By 1944, numerous local associations of blind people had formed in urban communities. How then to bring these together?

About a dozen such clubs were operating in Ontario, and attempts to organize them began in 1943 at a meeting in Toronto. In February 1944, a second meeting was held in London, Ontario, after the Manitoba League wrote to the London Association of the Blind suggesting a possible affiliation.

Attending that meeting in London was Gilbert Layton, son of CFOB and MAB founder Philip Layton. Gilbert Layton had taken over management of the MAB and

had been invited to attend because the CFOB had links with several of these associations. Joined at the meeting by two delegates from Manitoba, Layton proposed that the meeting adopt the CFOB constitution.

However, prior to the meeting, the London Association of the Blind and the Manitoba League had withdrawn from the CFOB, as had other groups, so there was no support to accept Layton's proposal, and the meeting decided on a separate constitution.

Although Baker did not attend this founding meeting, his fine hand was likely played by Arthur Magill, who was present as the CNIB administrator. Sadie Bending was elected as the first president, and William Johnson and Ivan Hunter were elected as vice-presidents of the new inter-provincial group, made up of Ontario and Manitoba, called the Canadian Council of the Blind.

Over the next three years, the CCB held meetings in Winnipeg, Halifax, and Vancouver. In Vancouver, the White Cane Club (formerly called Nil Desperandum, or "Do Not Despair") became the provincial affiliate.

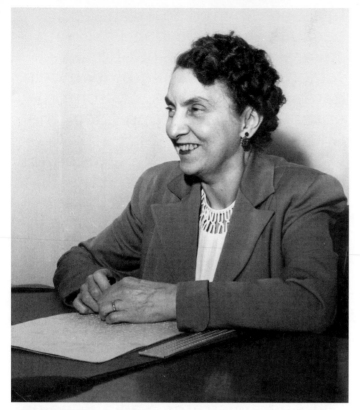

Sadie Bending, first president of the Canadian Council of the Blind (1944–1960).

CCB headquarters were established in London at the CNIB office, probably because Bending, who would serve as its president for sixteen years, lived in that city.

Based on the important precedent set earlier in Manitoba in 1920, the CNIB financed the CCB's activities, including travel, meetings, and conferences. Gradually, the CCB acquired national staff who were funded by the CNIB and who, until 1985, held CNIB employee status.

When it was founded, the CCB had obtained a federal charter and eventually formed provincial divisions that mirrored the CNIB divisions in structure. A contest was held to name their publication, and *CCB Outlook* was chosen as the winner.

Eventually, the CFOB gave up its efforts to compete with the CNIB at a national level, and the group fragmented into more provincial structures. By 1960, its strength was mostly aligned with the Montreal Association for the Blind, which had spawned and nurtured it.

Once the CFOB had been vanquished, or nearly so, Baker recognized the need for an alternative national association of the blind. He knew that similar associations of blind people, both war-blinded and civilian, were at work in other countries, and he astutely recognized in the early 1960s that an effective national consumer organization of the blind in Canada would be an important ally in pushing for public policies and legislation. He also saw a role for a consumer group in monitoring CNIB services and its clients' experiences with the institute.

Jacobus ten Broek, an Albertan who taught law at the University of California at Berkeley, had been instrumental in founding the National Federation of the Blind in the United States in 1940. Led by ten Broek and others in Europe and elsewhere, the International Federation of the Blind was formed in direct opposition to the World Council for the Welfare of the Blind that had been created in 1951 after two previous attempts in 1931 and 1948 had failed. After prolonged negotiations, the two international organizations of and for the blind united to form the World Blind Union in 1984. CNIB Managing Director Ross Purse and his successor, Robert Mercer, both attended the decisive merger summit in Antwerp, Belgium.

That historic evolution and the philosophy of "we, the blind, speaking for ourselves" led to the so-called consumer movement. To the uninitiated, the two prepositions "of" and "for" have taken on a new significance never to be reversed. An organization "for" the blind is generally run by well-meaning sighted people, while an organization "of" the blind is exactly that.

When the two types of organizations are in conflict, confusion in the public mind and a duplication of effort result. When philosophical or ideological differences develop, as happened often in Canada and other countries, the blind find themselves divided if not conquered; they are often marginalized or, worse, ignored. However, the experience of groups working together has demonstrated that much can be achieved. Had the CNIB and CFOB not spent thirty-odd years in open warfare, greater strides might well have been made sooner in improving the quality of life for the blind, including expanding employment opportunities.

To a lesser extent, there was also conflict among other consumer groups after 1960, and the public often found it difficult to differentiate among blindness organizations or to understand who they were and what they did.

RECREATION

Shortly after the CCB was formed, recreation became a priority. In

1948, and for the next ten years, the CCB and CNIB operated a summer camp at Ancaster, Ontario, near Hamilton, as a joint project.

As interest grew and participation increased, a larger facility was needed, and in 1962, a twelve-acre site on Lake Joseph, about 120 miles (200 kilometres) north of Toronto was chosen. The land had a romantic past: it had originally been used as a railway siding for overnight sleeping trains from Toronto carrying Muskoka cottage trade waiting to board the steamships that plied the Muskoka lakes ferrying the

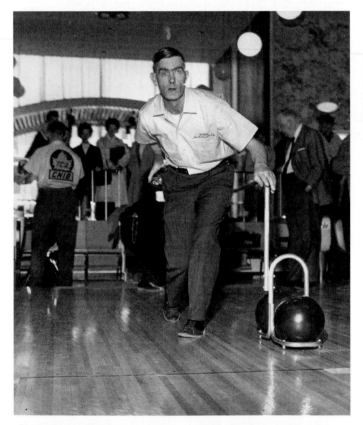

A special guide rail lets champion bowler George Mills from New Westminster, British Columbia, enjoy an afternoon at the lanes.

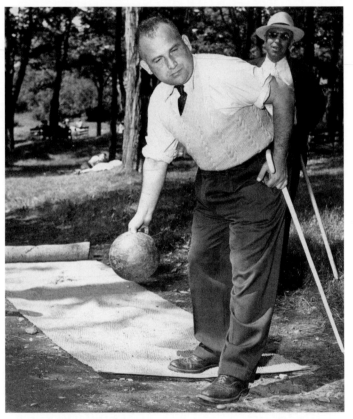

Lawn bowling was a popular summer pastime.

gentry to their summer cottages. The land was purchased from the Canadian National Railway for $25,000, and buildings were constructed with support from Lions Clubs and government grants. The Lions support has continued for over forty years, representing a huge financial contribution.

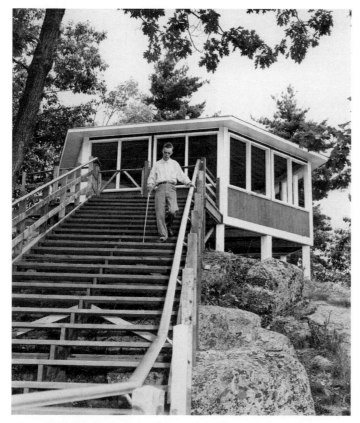

A camper at the Lake Joseph Holiday Centre makes his way down from Kentwood Point.

By 1981, costs and operating requirements of this 120-bed attractive facility, now known as the Lake Joseph Centre, were escalating. Responsibility for the centre, which provides priceless opportunities for disabled people of all ages to enjoy the recreational joys of summer, was taken over by the CNIB's Ontario division.

BOWEN ISLAND

It is generally accepted that a healthy rivalry existed between Baker and Captain M.C. Robinson, superintendent of the B.C.-Yukon division. That may account for the B.C.-Yukon division's decision to acquire land on Deep Cove, Bowen Island, in Horseshoe Bay just outside Vancouver. In September of 1961, the Union Steamship Company agreed to sell the three-acre wooded site, with its breathtaking view of Howe Sound and the coastal mountain range, for $50,000, less a donation of $10,000. An eleven-thousand-square foot lodge was erected at a cost of $155,169 and officially opened, with the provincial minister of recreation in attendance, in

183

May 1963. The facility provided accommodation for forty-four blind people and their escorts and offered a variety of summer sports and adjustment to blindness training courses.

A two-hundred-year-old totem pole, one of three that stood on Bowen Island, is perhaps the most symbolic presence and certainly the most visible tie between the CNIB and Canada's coastal Native populations. The pole was restored as part of the CNIB's seventy-fifth anniversary celebrations in 1993.

The CCB and CNIB also operated camps in Atlantic Canada, but none were owned outright. Over time, both Bowen Island and the Lake Joseph Centre sites became valuable land acquisitions, worth millions of dollars.

Besides offering blind people the chance to enjoy summer recreational activities in a safe, supported environment, the facili-

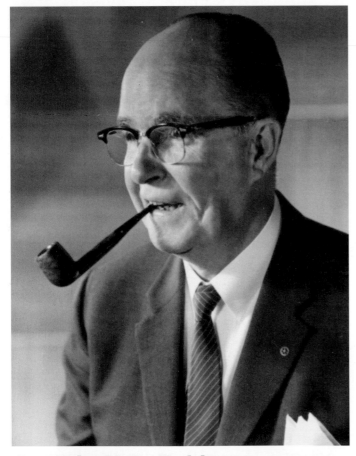

Captain M.C. Robinson, superintendent of the B.C.-Yukon division.

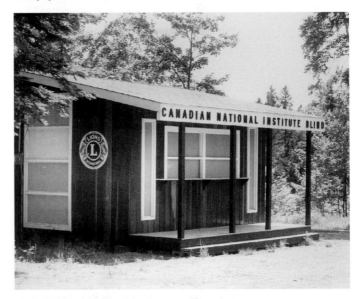

Coxheath was a summer camp run by the Lions Club near Sydney, Nova Scotia.

ties also gave blind teenagers and adults opportunities to socialize, meet potential partners, and form long-lasting friendships.

WHITE CANE WEEK

People who are blind have used sticks or canes as tools for travel for centuries. But it was not until 1921 that the white cane became the symbol of blindness. An English photographer who had lost his sight decided to use a white cane to let people in his community know he was blind.

In North America, the introduction of the white cane is attributed to Lions Clubs International. In 1930, a Lions Club member watched as a man who was blind attempted to cross the street with a black cane that was barely visible to motorists against the dark pavement. The Lions decided to paint the cane white to make it more visible. In 1931, the Lions Clubs International adopted the promotion of white canes for people who are blind as a national program.

Ivan Hunter from Windsor, who later became a CNIB staff member, is credited with introducing an annual public awareness educational program known as White Cane Week in 1946. This program, held each year during the first week of February, was a joint CNIB-CCB venture and was focused solely on education, with no fundraising component.

The week grew into a media success story with extensive outreach programs in schools, service clubs, and government sectors. The CCB, with few staff and even fewer financial resources, relied

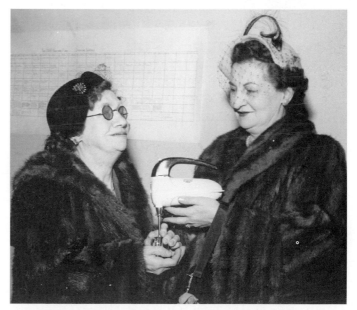

Norah Fall (left) first-prize winner of a White Cane Week cooking contest, receives her prize from Mrs. Allan Lamport, 1954.

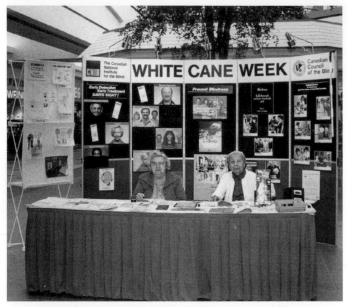

A White Cane Week mall display, Manitoba, 1988.

heavily on the CNIB from the outset to plan, brand, and execute the program. From the beginning, there was friction among individuals in both organizations. As White Cane Week grew, CNIB leadership was not always onside, and careful discussions had to take place to smooth ruffled feathers.

By the 1990s, CNIB management had grown tired of assigning their staff to perform a disproportionate share of the White Cane Week work and of having to pay for all the collateral materials (such as bookmarks, rulers, and buttons) that an awareness campaign, with a children's component, requires. Fundraising began to creep in around the week, and in 2003 the program was ceded to the CCB.

STERILIZATION

Policy and practice of sterilization with respect to disabled people and eugenics worldwide, including Canada, are far from fictional notions. In 2000, at the general assembly held in Melbourne, Australia, the World Blind Union, sponsored by the blind women's committee, adopted a policy reaffirming the right of blind and other disabled women to bear children without prejudice or legislative injunctions.

Sterilization of the blind was a serious issue facing the CNIB leadership in the 1930s.

In December of 1936, A.R. Kaufman, of Kitchener, Ontario, sent a brief letter to D.B. Lawley, the CNIB's Ontario district service manager, expressing his strongly held view that "all blind people who marry should have the privilege of exercising birth control either through contraceptives or preferable sterilization when there is any fear of congenital blindness or inability of the parents to support their children." Kaufman, who owned the Kaufman Rubber Co., offered through his organization, the Parents' Information Bureau, "to give free birth control information and contraceptive supplies to any blind people in Canada you may indicate, and I am also willing to attempt to make arrangements for the sterilization of blind people on your request."

Some months later, not having heard back from the CNIB, Kaufman wrote again, a longer letter this time:

> The day may come when your organization may have to take birth control measures more seriously for lack of funds to cope with results while ignoring what I think is the chief contributing cause to the difficulties of the blind. I hope you will not interpret my letter to mean that I have no sympathy for the blind. I think I have far more practical sympathy than your organization, or you would do something more constructive than merely trying to care for people who wish they had never been born.

Kaufman went on to describe, in very emotional language, a blind acquaintance of his who had requested sterilization:

> I do not know how your Board feels about it but our blind friend cannot see any justice in raising innocent children doomed to blindness who have a right to resent such inheritance. I do not think our friend would change his mind even if you assured him you would look after his children. I do not think the care you would give is sufficient compensation to the children for being born with the threatened handicap of blindness and all the grief that goes with it.

Kaufman then stated that he expected to receive a reply to his letter from the secretary of the CNIB.

By December 1938, Kaufman, having received no satisfactory response from the CNIB, wrote once again, this time directly to CNIB Managing Director Edwin Baker, explaining why voluntary sterilization of blind people was to be encouraged. His letter was forceful and blunt:

> I do not understand how the Canadian National Institute for the Blind can ignore sterilization … If you feel that you are going to invite complications by taking any active part in the sterilization of blind people, I suggest you send the names to me without any further comment. I have facilities to arrange sterilizations and since my Bureau has had blind people sterilized without your co-operation, it will likely be easier still if we get the names from you. You, of course, understand that all sterilizations are voluntary and we do not wish it otherwise, as we have our hands full enough with those who are anxiously waiting for sterilization.
>
> I hope to hear from you by letter stating the opinion of your Board on the question of sterilization [and] I will appreciate knowing the approximate percentage of your patients who are afflicted with congenital blindness.

Finally, almost two years to the day since Kaufman first wrote the CNIB, after a gracious apology for not replying sooner, Baker told him what he wanted to hear.

> You have asked for an opinion from the National Council of this Institute. This subject has not been discussed before and I cannot, on their behalf at this time, express an opinion with regard to sterilization. I can, however, express personal views.

To my knowledge, there has been no opposition throughout our Institute to sterilization … In fact, the special cases where their blindness is due to a hereditary condition and whom we knew sufficiently well to broach the subject, we have encouraged sterilization either before or as soon as possible after marriage.

While he emphasized that "any suggestion for the general sterilization of the blind would meet with my active and strenuous opposition," Baker carefully summed up his remarks by saying, "where any blind person's loss of sight was ophthalmologically certified as due to hereditary conditions or social disease which might, in any way, be transmitted to offspring, I would heartily support sterilization."

Within the year, Baker had authorized the CNIB district board in Brockville, Ontario, to cover the costs of having four blind men sterilized.

At the time, sterilization was generally accepted worldwide as an acceptable practice in cases of congenital defects.

LEGISLATING CHANGE

At local and federal levels, the CCB lobbied for legislative changes and travel and other concessions for blind people. Paramount in their campaign was the introduction of the hard reality that extraordinary costs are associated with blindness. The group also provided feedback to the CNIB on the quality of its services and suggested what CNIB priorities should be. A group known as the liaison committee met at least annually for a formal exchange of information and views.

The combined force of the two national organizations offered a common front to seek legislative changes. After a fourteen-year advocacy campaign championed by Baker, an act providing for pensions for blind people was passed by the Canadian Parliament on March 22, 1937, as an amendment to the Old Age Pensions Act, making the provisions of the act applicable to blind people at the age of forty, instead of seventy. The maximum pension was $20 per month, just the same as the old age pension, but blind pensioners were entitled to receive more earnings than was an old age pensioner before the amount of their pension would be affected. A single man or woman was entitled to receive a pension of $240 a year and was permitted to earn $200 a year before any deduction would be made. Provisions were also made for married couples.

The disability tax credit (DTC) originated during the Second World War as a $480 deduction from taxable income for people who were totally blind and did not claim an amount for attendant care under the medical expense deduction. This provision was intended to recognize undocumented, non-discretionary costs that blind people usually incur and to help compensate unpaid family members involved in their care.

A more recent example of successful lobbying came in the early 1990s with the introduction of the Goods and Services (GST) tax; the CNIB is cited in the legislation to assure exemption from the GST on low-vision devices, adaptive technology, and other items imported for the benefit and use of blind people.

As early as 1921, the city of Toronto issued permits that exempted a blind person from paying transit fares, and eventually other cities followed suit, offering free transit or a reduced fare. Also in the 1920s, Canadian National Railways offered a two-for-one tariff so a companion, who would act as a guide, could travel with a blind person. Theatre chains offered free entry on a weekly basis, and in British Columbia, Woodward Department Stores offered a discount to its blind customers.

On July 1, 1927, the forerunner to the Canadian Broadcasting Corporation celebrated Canada's sixtieth birthday with a coast-to-coast radio hookup. As a concession to blind people, the five-dollar license fee for a radio was waived. For blind people, many of whom were receiving information over the airwaves for the first time, this was empowerment. Recognizing the importance of broadcast communication as a tiny step toward independence, long before the audio book was introduced, the CNIB supplied radios to some clients for fifty years. (The organization also distributed used clothing, coal, glasses, and sometimes cash. This reflected living conditions in the 1920s and '30s.)

In 1935, in various cities across Canada, 17,952 passes to motion picture theatres and thousands of street car passes were distributed, most of them through CNIB offices.

The concessions were of enormous importance to blind people, given that the majority of them had a low standard of living, and statutory provisions for the blind came long before provisions for other civilian disabled Canadians.

The federal government passed the Blind Persons Act in 1948, and several provinces followed with acts called the Blind Persons' Rights Act or the White Cane Act. These acts made it a punishable offence for anyone who was not registered with the CNIB to carry or use a white cane, and later amendments included provisions guaranteeing a blind person the right to be accompanied by a specially trained guide dog in all public accommodations. These and other provisions came about as a direct result of the advocacy and lobbying by the two organizations.

In 2004, Her Honour Lois Hole, lieutenant governor of Alberta, proclaimed the Blind Persons' Rights Amendment Act, which was the result of the CNIB hard at work in Alberta.

The amendment act included many important improvements to the old Blind Persons' Rights Act, including the removal of any reference to the CNIB, a change in the way a blind person is described, and increases in fines.

In the old act, a blind person was defined as, "a person who is registered as blind with the Canadian National Institute for the Blind, or who, on account of blindness, receives a pension from the Government of Alberta, or who is certified by a qualified eye specialist as having not more than 6/60 vision ..." This was replaced by the much simpler, "a person who is blind according to accepted medical standards ..."

The amendment also raised the fine for any person other than a blind person carrying or using a white cane in a public place to $250 from $25; any person purporting to be blind for the purpose of claiming a benefit covered under the act could be fined $300, up from $100; and anyone denying a blind person accommodation or services to which the public is customarily admitted for the reason that the blind person was accompanied by a guide dog could face a fine of $3,000.

The amendment also extended to guide dogs in training and their trainers the same protection under the act as a blind person and a guide dog.

The Copyright Act amendment, passed in 1997, was another landmark achievement. After ten years of lobbying, the CNIB Library for the Blind became exempt from copyright law, which gave it the right to produce material in braille, e-text, or audio for the personal use of blind people.

Voting with privacy has also evolved slowly with a wide range of practices over the years. By the early 1980s blind voters had gained a measure of personal independence through the use of templates, which they could use to mark their ballots.

Until very recently, the district returning officer or a friend or family member had to read the candidates' names, and, depending on the number, the blind voter then had to memorize them, in order, so he would know where to mark the template. In a municipal election where as many as forty people could be running for positions on city council and boards of education, this system is at best awkward, and at worst patently unfair and discriminatory. Blind voters may also have a sworn witness mark their ballot for them. While braille ballots are not available, officials can sometimes offer information on voting procedures in braille, although that is rare.

In some jurisdictions, electronic voting has recently become more common, but regrettably, no common standard or practice has yet been introduced. Elections Canada, and most provinces, however, have been proactive, and by the 1990s they seemed to have understood that the ability to cast a vote in private is essential in a modern democracy and a basic right to which all voters, blind, visually impaired, or sighted, are entitled. Continuing pressure on Elections Canada will be necessary to bring about a seamless procedure when blind people vote.

But not all legislation favoured blind people. Acts governing jury duty, for example, prohibit a blind person from serving as a juror. This discriminatory practice, which seems based on ancient prejudices equating sight with intelligence, remains an issue in practice if not in law. The media have also been responsible for perpetuating this concept, often using blindfolded politicians in editorial cartoons to symbolize stupidity, or making gratuitous references to blindness.

CCB WANES

Over time, the CCB grew to include more than ninety local affiliates that seemed to focus on social and recreational activities. National tournaments for blind people who enjoyed card games, bowling, and curling were held annually. The CCB's efforts predated blind sports organizations and the Para Olympics; their tournaments were always well organized and well attended.

The CCB also worked tirelessly to pressure the Bank of Canada into introducing bank notes specially marked with raised dots so blind people could differentiate among denominations. After much consultation, the notes were introduced to Canadians in 2001. The CCB also worked with the Royal Mint on the creation of identifiable coins.

Every two years the CCB held a large convention at which resolutions were adopted.

Eventually, however, times changed, and two major developments contributed to the CCB's decline, which began in the 1980s. In the 1960s, other consumer organizations began to emerge, and these began to attract younger blind people who were not interested in what the staid CCB had to offer. The CCB's role in recreation began to wane as blind youth ventured into ice hockey, swimming, skiing, and adapted sports such as goal ball.

While a national organization for parents of blind children never materialized, other national groups had emerged by the 1980s. The National Federation of the Blind: Advocates for Equality, the Christian-based John Milton Society for the Blind, and blind sports groups were all launched.

At the same time, organizations like the Council for Canadians with Disabilities had strong national voices, and many blind individuals chose to affiliate with these emerging groups.

The fact that the CCB was wholly funded by the CNIB did, over time, diminish its credibility as an independent consumer organization; it was often said that the CCB was nothing more than a mouthpiece for the CNIB. This accusation was grossly unfair to each organization.

After the CNIB's financial support to the CCB was phased out over a five-year period from about 1984 to 1989, staff were formally transferred to the CCB and offices were relocated to Ottawa from London. From that point, the organization struggled to regain its former structure, membership, and effectiveness.

The national operation of the CCB was left near penniless and without a functioning fundraising program. The CCB divisions and individual clubs do have financial resources, but there has been no willingness to share the wealth to preserve the integrity and influence of the national body.

To suggest, with hindsight, that the CNIB's role in the formation and support of the CCB was a failed experiment would be inaccurate. However, the approach was unsound from the beginning because it created dependency. The CNIB retained bottom line control of an annual budget of some $500,000, including what was funded by the operating divisions.

As CCB membership began to fall off, the clubs turned to CNIB staff who had confidential knowledge of new clients to refer these potential members to them; despite sporadic membership drives, more and more of the CNIB's new clients were simply not interested in joining.

In many areas, CCB clubs clustered around CNIB residential facilities that were gradually being phased out. The CCB's membership dwindled, and the leadership seldom changed. The weakening of the CCB's influence and reach meant that the CNIB could ignore consumer responses from this group. The diminishing of the CCB also reduced the ability of blind Canadians to speak with one forceful voice at national and international levels.

Given the CNIB's size and scope as a service organization with significant resources, a truly independent and financially viable consumer organization able to hold the organization to account to the blind of Canada, its most important stakeholders, would probably have been a good thing.

CHAPTER 9
The Years of Expansion

When the Second World War broke out in September 1939, the CNIB, along with the rest of the country, had been catching its breath from the financial struggles and hardship of the Great Depression. Meeting payrolls and paying suppliers had been a constant worry.

The intervening years from the organization's founding in 1918 had been a time of slow and methodical progress, with some spectacular successes.

The CNIB was well organized, with two divisions in Western Canada, one in the Maritimes, and one in Quebec; as well, the national office operated programs in Ontario. The library, along with several departments for training and administration, was working well. The nerve centre of the CNIB, at 186 Beverley Street, was humming. General Manager Arthur V. Weir and Managing Director Edwin Baker controlled the levers of power, aided by two senior managers designated to oversee operations in Eastern and Western

Canada. Dr. John MacDonald, superintendent from the time the division opened until his death in 1946, was responsible for the vast area of Quebec to the East Coast, while Captain M.C. Robinson was responsible for Manitoba to the Pacific Ocean. MacDonald was never replaced, and Robinson retained the courtesy title National Director of Western Canada until his retirement in 1964.

Workshops provided jobs in at least ten cities, and four residences — one each in Ottawa and Hamilton and two in Toronto — provided care and safe, comfortable accommodation to blind people. Smaller facilities in residential houses dotted several communities in other provinces. Economic security for the average blind person had improved with the introduction of the pension in 1937, and by 1948 the Blind Persons Act had been adopted.

In 1958, the eligibility age for the pension was lowered to eighteen, and the monthly allowance, subject to a means test, was increased to $75. The CNIB had introduced a national identification card system assigning client registration numbers, which were needed to gain access to travel, theatre, tax credits, and other concessions.

The registration number program remains in effect to this day, although other means to qualify blind people for certain services was broadened somewhat in the 1980s, authorizing certain professions or individuals to validate a blind person's entitlement. For blind people, CNIB registration is generally accepted as valid identification, in lieu of a driver's licence or other documentation, and proof of eligibility for reduced fares. The accounting and cash flow structure of the CNIB allowed it to move surplus funds from one program to another or from one part of Canada to another as need arose, and income from the canteen program and workshops was managed this way. This system is no small feature within the CNIB and is almost without precedent in Canadian philanthropy.

Operating the national office and the Ontario division as one entity simplified matters and made Baker's life much easier because most of the money funding the organization was coming from Ontario in general, and Toronto specifically, until 1950.

Field personnel were obtaining donations from service clubs and women's organizations, holding local campaigns, such as the popular "tag days," and organizing door-to-door solicitations. Many of these staff members had been trained by David Lawley, national consultant of field services, in the fundamentals of fundraising.

From thirty years of experience, National Council President Lew Wood and Baker knew that

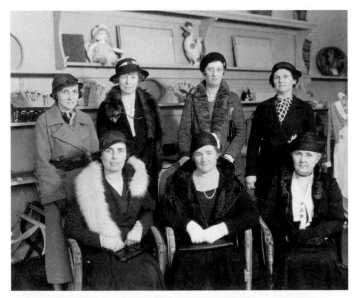

Tag Day advisory board, 1933. Front row (left to right): Elsinore Burns, Lady Baillie, Mrs. Lionel Clarke. Back row (left to right): Mrs. Melville Grant, Mrs. R.L. Merry, Miss Jean Wood, Mrs. Percy Henderson.

the best way to raise money for the CNIB was to recruit influential men and women and high-profile business leaders within their own communities. Business Manager Weir's quiet "slow speaking, deep thinking" and steady influence anchored their efforts.

This early model of fundraising and awareness strategy works just as well today. As a blind veteran in a leadership position, Baker had easy access to top officials in Ottawa. Occasional appointments with the prime minister of the day ensured that his requests were heard and considered at the highest level. As blind veterans obtained pensions and benefits, the spillover was felt by other blind Canadians. For example, although preference would be given to a blind veteran to operate a retail kiosk in a federal building, if no suitable blind veteran was available, the CNIB could fill the position with a civilian.

Shortly after Canada entered the war, Baker was quick to tell the federal government that the CNIB was in a strong position to accept and rehabilitate veterans who might lose their sight in the war effort. This time, there was no competition or duplication of efforts with the Montreal Association for the Blind or the Halifax School, as had been the case during the First World War. The government agreed, and Harvey Lyons, a First World War veteran, was posted to England as part of the after-care service team available to wounded Canadians. Once identified, rather than having to take rehabilitation courses in England, as had been the case in 1915, the men were returned home to Canada, where training awaited them in Toronto.

In the fall of 1943, the wealthy Lady Virginia Kemp, widow of sheet metal baron Sir Edward Kemp, purchased a large house at 186 Admiral Road in Toronto. The house was remodelled and furnished by Lady Kemp's daughter, Katherine, and on March 23, 1944, His Excellency the Earl of Athlone, Governor General of Canada, accompanied by Her Royal Highness, Princess Alice, formally presented the house, named Baker Hall, to the CNIB.

Over the course of the Second World War and beyond, approximately 125 blinded servicemen, 25 to 30 at a time, resided at Baker

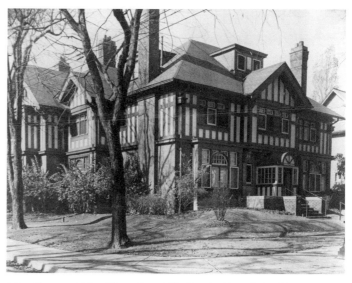

Baker Hall at 186 Admiral Road in Toronto, the gift of Lady Kemp.

Hall while they took rehabilitation courses at Pearson Hall. Their stay in the program would last up to nine months.

Elwood Greenfield was recruited from the Ontario School for the Blind in 1946 to teach braille to the veterans at Pearson Hall. The first male rehabilitation teacher, Greenfield completed the CNIB training in 1950, after which he went on to have a most distinguished career in Saskatoon, serving clients in northern Saskatchewan. Later in his working life he headed a group that wrote a book, published only in braille, called *50 Years of Rehabilitation Teaching in Canada*. Following their rehabilitation, many of the men went on to higher education, entered professions, and pursued successful careers. Others met the women they would marry at the social events, like tea dances, organized for them at Baker Hall.

Home teachers, social workers, and volunteers rallied to this remarkable effort. Elizabeth Rusk, Lady Kemp, and Elsinore Burns are a few of the many women who played a prominent role in what is truly a wonderful success story. In all, about fifteen rehabilitation staff members worked with the Baker Hall veterans to help them regain their independence. Baker Hall was sold in 1952, and the proceeds were used as a trust fund to help blind individuals.

Lady Kemp's long association with the CNIB had begun in 1927 when she joined the Toronto Women's Auxiliary. She became its president in 1934, a post she held until 1945. In 1939 she was chosen vice-president of the institute, and in 1954 she assumed the presidency, taking over from Lewis M. Wood, who had been the presi-dent since the CNIB's founding in 1918. She resigned in 1957 because of ill health and was made an honorary president.

At the time Lady Kemp assumed the presidency, the CNIB was serving twenty thousand clients from forty-seven service centres and offices across Canada. About thirty-five rehabilitation teachers were on staff. Admired throughout her life for her great beauty and respected for her end-less philanthropy, Lady Kemp, one of Toronto's last titled gentle-women, died after a short illness in June 1957.

The week before she died she had given a garden party at her home, Castle Frank, for the war-blinded members of the Sir Arthur Pearson Association and their wives. One of the last luncheon parties at her home was given in honour of Helen Keller. The young men who benefited so greatly from Lady Kemp's generosity, returning from prisoner of war camps in Europe and the Far East, far out-numbered the relatively few men who had trickled back from the First World War.

The program proved to be a fertile recruiting ground as the

CNIB was able to draw from this group of newly trained and educated veterans. Some were offered positions in management while others worked in catering, field service, or administration. Ross C. Purse, who went on to become managing director of the CNIB in 1973, and William Mayne, who also had a long and distinguished career with CNIB, had lost their sight while incarcerated as prisoners of war in the Far East. Both were rehabilitated at Baker Hall and then recruited by the CNIB when they returned to their homes in Manitoba.

THE BUILDING BOOM

The post-war economy saw CNIB operations and programs expand at a remarkable pace. The leadership went into high gear in every province. The industrial programs had grown to large commercial operations, and fundraising had become almost an art form. Governments were receptive to appeals from the institute to offer incentive grants for services and capital growth.

Two major construction programs followed. Residences that also served as service centres integrated a new design and concept from previous buildings. Planning was well underway by 1954 for a bold and imaginative campus to be built at 1929 Bayview Avenue in Toronto. Arthur Magill, who had been seconded to the United Nations in 1953 to oversee the construction of a rehabilitation centre in the Middle East, was recalled to Toronto to help with the $3.5-million capital campaign for the land acquisition and construction costs.

County houses in Ontario had been described by the newly hired Magill in 1936 as "much like Elizabethan poor houses and homes for the friendless." The living conditions, he said, were appalling. Decent accommodation for blind people, who, for whatever reason, were unable to live with caring family members or who were aging was rare. For some blind people, the county houses were the only option.

A feature of the Canadian landscape as a matter of public policy spanning at least one hundred years from 1860 was the construction of massive facilities strategically located in each province as a form of hospital or hospice built to essentially warehouse a sizable sector of the population considered "mentally ill, criminally insane, retarded" or disabled.

An unconscionable number of blind adults found themselves living in these awful warehouses, alongside people considered mentally ill, low functioning, or multi-disabled. Blind people were sometimes misdiagnosed or labelled as low-performing, high-risk patients, and blindness was often considered a disability requiring institutionalization. Once the elements of blindness were understood and specific remedial care was provided, the option of living in the community returned.

To partly resolve these needs, affecting an estimated 10 percent of the registered blind in Ontario, the CNIB decided to build ten residences in key urban locations, including Sudbury in the north and Thunder Bay in the northwest. These new residences would be in addition to the ones that already existed.

These buildings were no longer just residences but became hubs for service and social activities. A blind resident, male or female,

was now afforded a standard of living and comfort that many had never known. On August 23, 1948, Linwell Hall, which had been built at a cost of $120,000, opened in St. Catharines, followed within weeks by a new facility in Saskatoon. In 1949 the Lions Residence in Winnipeg welcomed its first residents.

By 1964, there were three facilities in B.C., two each in Alberta and Saskatchewan, one each in Quebec City and Saint John, and two in Newfoundland (in Cornerbrook and St. John's). The Quebec City residence, built in 1964, was the last to open.

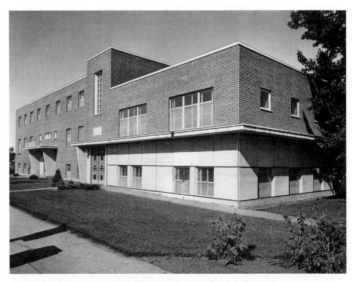

Northern Alberta Service Centre and Residence, Jasper Avenue, Edmonton, Alberta.

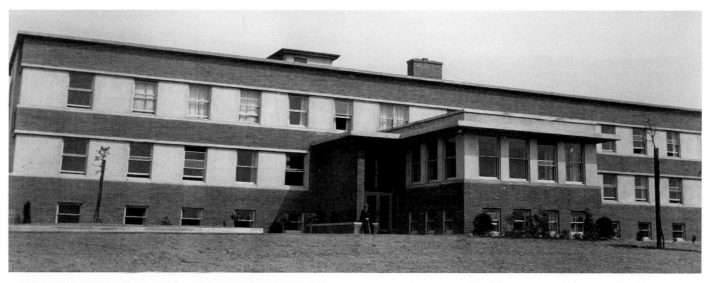

Queen Elizabeth Hall in Vancouver was built in 1950. A new wing was added in 1955.

Ironically, as it accepted its first residents, vacancies were already becoming a concern in other parts of Canada.

No residence was opened in Halifax as the management and board held the firm view not to have a residence as a matter of principle. No evidence was found to suggest that the Maritime division's decision to not construct residences in Nova Scotia and Prince Edward Island was ever at variance with national office or the other provincial divisions, all of which operated residential programs for about fifty years. One explanation could be that Division Superintendent Frank Flinn and Baker were close associates, and Baker was a frequent visitor to the Flinn home on his trips to Halifax.

Capital campaigns to raise money were supplemented by government grants. Surplus operating funds from the industrial programs were also directed toward financing these buildings, which, at their height, numbered at least twenty-five, plus the two summer camps. Short-term mortgages were obtained in a few instances but were retired quickly.

Donations of furniture and kitchen and office equipment provided opportunities for "named

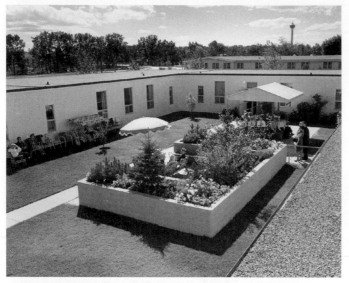

Residence and garden, 1260 Memorial Drive East, Calgary.

gifts" from individuals, service clubs, and women's groups. A plaque in Clarkewood, the residence in Toronto, reads, "Clarkewood Residence for the Blind officially opened by His Excellency the Rt. Hon. Vincent Massey, CH, Governor General of Canada on April 16, 1956" and credits the J.P. Bicknell Foundation for providing furniture and equipment. Similar plaques, with the names changed to fit the circumstances, could be found in every CNIB building throughout Canada. They were later replaced by a more contemporary design, referred to as "donor walls."

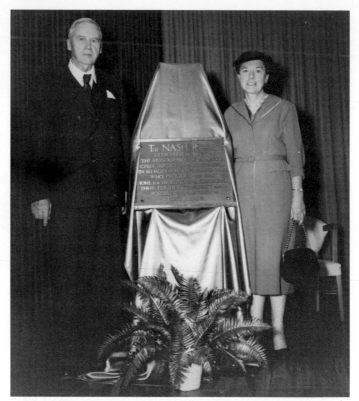

The Honourable W.H. Martin, chief justice of Saskatchewan, with Marjorie Rollefson, granddaughter of T. Frank Nash, at the dedication of the CNIB Nash Residence, Regina, Saskatchewan, 1955.

By the 1950s, donated cars, mostly from Lions clubs, provided transportation for the residence and the field staff, who until then had relied on public transportation.

It's worth noting that these service centres, often constructed on prime land, were highly visible and modern, and the communities took pride in them. Land values could only increase, as indeed they did!

Heightened community interest brought with it new volunteers and donations of food, which supplemented the operating budget. A new stream of income also emerged in the form of bequests as auxiliary members included the institute or residence in their wills.

In Toronto, meanwhile, the CNIB's operations were scattered across five locations, mostly in the downtown core. Separate residences existed for men and women, who were also segregated in their workshops. Relocations took place as more space was needed. Early on, the Beverley Street site had been expanded as demands on the national office increased and the number of staff grew. Office space, however, became so cramped that at some point the switchboard was installed on a staircase landing.

The inevitability of a major relocation from Pearson Hall reached its climax by the late 1940s. It was at this juncture, pressured by volunteers and staff from outside Toronto, that the decision was made to separate the Ontario division from the national office to clarify the roles and status of Ontario staff and volunteers.

Arthur Napier Magill was appointed the third superintendent of the Ontario division, which came back into being after a thirty-year gap. The separation of powers and function begged the question on how to finance the national office. A funding formula was eventually agreed upon: each division was assessed an amount based on its gross operating budget. The exception was Ontario, which was given the privilege of paying double the amount of assessment.

BAKERWOOD

In June 1951, Baker advised his board that the time had come for the CNIB to have a purpose-built home of its own in which national headquarters and all of the Ontario division would be combined on one property with a new building, at a cost of about $1 to $1.5 million. Over the course of the next year, the Ontario division was established and property on Bayview Avenue was located and visited by council. Negotiating with the federal government's Department of Veterans Affairs, the CNIB purchased some ten acres of land that had been part of the Kilgour Estate, adjacent to Sunnybrook Hospital on what was then the northern edge of Toronto. In addition, a vacant lot at the corner of Bayview and Glenvale was purchased from the Toronto and York Roads Commission.

Throughout 1953 and 1954 a capital campaign was held to raise money for the new building. By September 1954, the campaign had reached $3.1 million with $1.4 million in pledges. In January 1956, the building was in move-in condition and the CNIB proudly opened its new campus, called BakerWood after co-founders Edwin Baker and Lewis Wood. The facility was state of the art for accessibility by the standards of the day. The four buildings that made up the campus covered some 1.8 hectares for a total of 15,000 square metres of space. The building was officially opened on April 16, 1956, when the Right Honourable Vincent Massey,

Governor General of Canada, passed the key to CNIB President Lady Kemp.

The building, which housed administration offices, the library, recreation facilities, workshops, a 140-bed residence, and catering facilities where meals for 800 people were prepared every day, was impressive and soon became a welcome Toronto landmark. Fronting Bayview Avenue to the west was the administration building with the familiar clock tower and facade.

An auditorium stood just to the north, with the library, cafeteria, and residence immediately behind. The large broom shop, warehouse, and packaging area were located on the lower level. An underground passageway allowed workshop personnel to travel safely from the Bayview Avenue bus stop to their work site. On this same level at the front of the building were well-stocked recreational facilities, including an exercise room and driving range.

On the second floor, as part of the clock tower, the stately boardroom was located. Named in honour of Lady Virginia Kemp, the room featured three large oil paint-

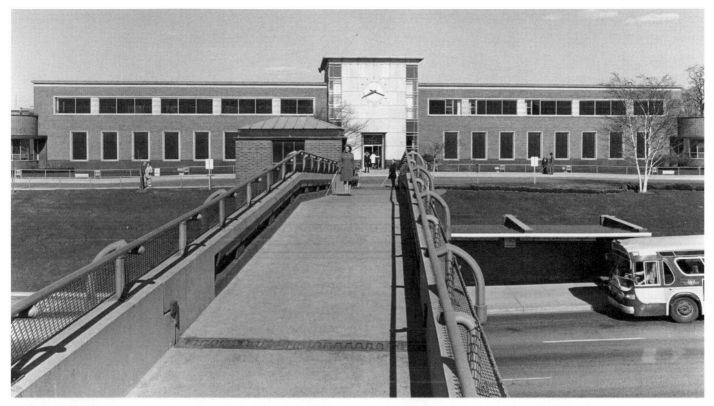

The bridge over Bayview Avenue leading to BakerWood, Toronto. The bridge was later enclosed.

ings of Edwin Baker and national presidents Lewis Wood and Lady Kemp, who gazed down benignly for two generations at the proceedings taking place around the massive boardroom table until the building was demolished in 2003.

Another familiar feature of the BakerWood site is the unique pedestrian overpass on Bayview Avenue, which was constructed on land owned by the institute bordering on Bayview Avenue and funded by the Atkinson Foundation.

Imagine some six hundred to eight hundred staff, residents, workshop employees, volunteers, administrators, the CaterPlan business, and a large, bustling library operation all working together in one location. For Canadians, this was the headquarters of their CNIB, and for international visitors it was a showcase facility.

Retail space for a gift shop and the sale of Blindcraft items drew in the public, and tours of the building were popular. At the front of the building, overlooking Bayview Avenue, a quiet, tastefully decorated room, reminiscent of a comfortable lounge in a gentlemen's club, was dedicated "in perpetuity" for the use of members of the Sir Arthur Pearson Association of War Blinded. This room, known as the SAPA Lounge, was opened only on rare, formal occasions, and annual Remembrance Day observances were held there. The SAPA Lounge cemented the CNIB's relationship with its past, reflecting a common heritage with Canada's war-blinded and the high regard in which the CNIB has always held them.

In the 1990s, Joanne MacKie, an assistant in the president's office, undertook to research the history of the CNIB's role in assisting the war-blinded, and the walls of the SAPA Lounge, through chronologically arranged photographs, plaques, citations, and other memorabilia, told the story. An audio guide to the room was also created.

The room also ensured that Sir Arthur Pearson and his founding association with the CNIB would not be forgotten when Pearson Hall, at 186 Beverley Street, was sold. Other parts of the building were used for pleasure. In one small room a ham radio shack was opened; across Canada more than four hundred blind ham radio operators and an equal number of sighted sponsors enjoyed keeping

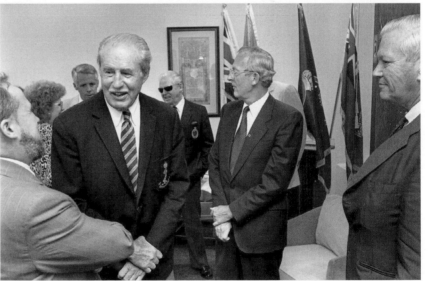

(Left to right) Euclid Herie, the Honourable George Hees, Tim Sheeres, and John Baker following the signing of a contract between Veterans Affairs Canada and the CNIB, early 1980s.

in touch with people all around the world — and this long before the days of e-mail and the Internet.

The buildings were set in spectacular parkland. The Toronto Garden Club, inspired by one of

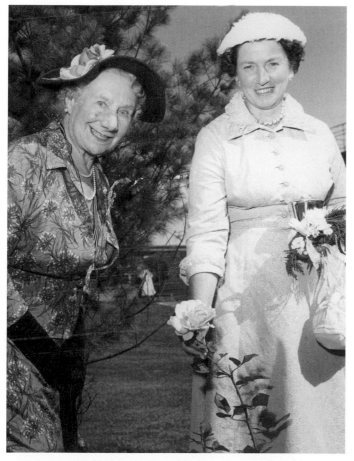

Muriel Paxman of the Colchester Rose Society (left) and Mrs. J.R.M. Wilson, chairman of the Fragrant Garden Committee, the Garden Club of Toronto, 1956.

Canada's most prominent gardeners of her day, Lois Wilson, designed and planted a world-class fragrant garden that would appeal to all the senses as the centrepiece of the facility. The garden, which came to be admired throughout Toronto as a beautiful, tranquil oasis, featured unique plantings selected for their properties to bring beauty to blind people. Some plants were chosen because they were highly fragranced, others for their texture, still others because they attract birds who would be welcome in the garden for their song. The names of all plants were posted in braille, and fountains with running water provided a soothing audio backdrop. The garden even featured a beautiful oak tree, a gift from Queen Elizabeth II, grown from an acorn taken from Windsor Great Park. There were generous seating arrangements with benches and chairs. Many plants were grown in raised beds so blind people would find it easier to stop and smell them, and the winding paths had raised edges to make navigating through the garden with a white cane easier. For fifty years, the garden brought much pleasure

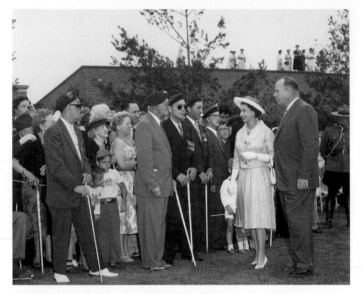

The queen, escorted by CNIB President Ralph Misener, meets members of the Sir Arthur Pearson Association for War Blinded during a walkabout in the Fragrant Garden, June 1959.

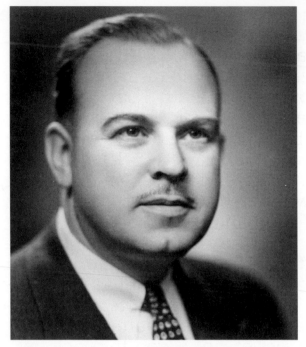

Ralph Misener.

to blind and sighted CNIB staff and volunteers, and other gardens around the world, including one in Capetown, South Africa, were modelled after it.

As Toronto grew, BakerWood didn't seem so far from downtown Toronto after all, and the site, with its distinctive overpass, became a familiar part of the city's streetscape.

In the 1960s, a small parcel of land to the east was severed and sold to two rehabilitation facilities. The CNIB retained 6.5 hectares of land bordering on a ravine. This masterful, visionary campus served the CNIB well for forty-eight years until the decision was made in 2002 to replace it with a new eleven-thousand-square-metre facility on a smaller parcel of land at the same location. The new building opened in 2004.

Elsewhere in Canada, the 1950s was also a period of rapid growth for the CNIB; the high-visibility building program in Toronto was repeated in almost every provincial capital. A service centre was built on Almon Street in Halifax, and the CNIB provided service in Charlottetown from a house on Grafton Street in the city centre. Fredericton did not acquire a building until much later.

In Ottawa, the CNIB occupied a large building on O'Connor Street, owned by the Ottawa Association of the Blind, which predated the formation of the CNIB. Here, an office, residence, and workshop were housed. The auditorium was called Letson Hall, after First World War veteran (and later client) Harry Letson. Given the location and high visibility of this building in the nation's capital, many people would have assumed it to be the national headquarters of the CNIB. Periodically there were thoughts that it would be desirable to locate the national office in Ottawa, but in fact the O'Connor Street building always served as a district operation for Ontario.

With few exceptions, every facility was fully financed within a reasonable time period. The financial challenge, demanding a shrewd budgeting process, was to generate the ballooning annual operating costs needed to maintain

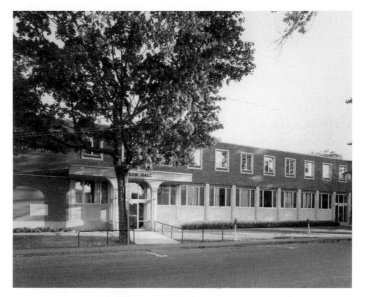

Letson Hall, residence and service centre, Ottawa.

these facilities. To that end, each operating division recruited a business manager to oversee its business and administrative operations. Services were directed by the superintendent, later known as the executive director, or if the demands of the centre were great enough in a particular location, by a field manager, later known as a district manager.

Each division had a board of management, and each district had an advisory board. In Ontario there were as many as eighty-nine advisory boards and committees comprised of three thousand members. The field personnel had increased to twenty-five to support the work. All were blind men; women would not be appointed for another eight or so years (with the exception of Mrs. J.F. Purvis, who is listed as the representative in Ottawa in 1936). Seventy-five other boards were in place throughout the country. Also busy in the service of the CNIB were several thousand more volunteers who served as visitors, drivers, fundraisers, braillists, audio transcribers, members of women's auxiliaries, and talking book repairmen, including the Telephone Pioneers — the level of activity was hectic.

THE A.V. WEIR CENTRE

The grand finale to this twenty-year building boom was the erection of the A.V. Weir Centre on Bayview Avenue, a national training and vocational guidance centre that was officially opened in 1968, the institute's fiftieth anniversary, by His Excellency Roland Michener, Governor General of Canada.

The building was named after Arthur V. Weir, a man with acute

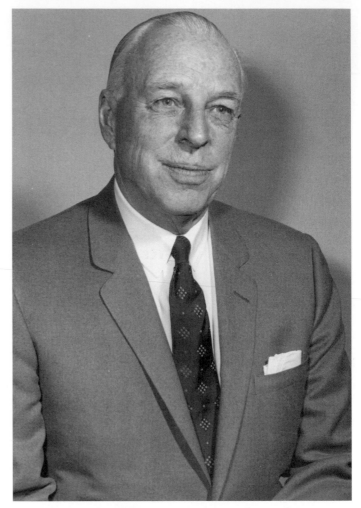

Arthur V. Weir, general manager of the CNIB.

business acumen who made an enormous contribution to the CNIB. He joined the institute in 1924 as business manager and served as general manager from 1942 until his retirement in 1964, working alongside Baker for forty-

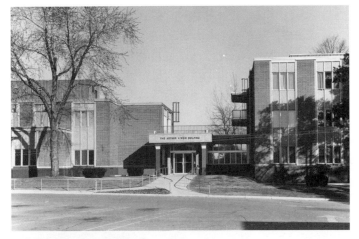

The A.V. Weir Centre.

one years. He was a quiet, gentle person who brought wisdom, competence, strength, and stability to the organization's accounting and business operations. Other than Baker, Weir is the only CNIB employee to be honoured by having a building named after him, a tribute that speaks volumes about the high regard in which the man and his contributions were held.

John Baker, son of Edwin Baker, described Weir as having provided the balance at the office that allowed his father the freedom to promote and direct the institute's affairs. In some respects, this close teamwork set a management model for operating divisions that served the CNIB well, given the level and scope of business activities, including management of real estate holdings and building projects.

At the time of Weir's retirement in 1964, the CNIB operated fifty offices across Canada, including twenty residences and service centres, and assisted more than twenty-five thousand blind men, women, and children — and Weir was credited with being a key factor in those achievements.

Blind veterans from both world wars had received structured and focused rehabilitation training at Pearson Hall. For the civilian blind, however, rehabilitation services were available inconsistently and sporadically in the early years.

With the opening of the A.V. Weir Centre and similar programs being offered in the divisions the two streams of clients — war-blinded and civilian — were now on a level playing field for rehabilitation training. The A.V. Weir Centre was at the leading edge of rehabilitation in the blindness field. The CNIB management had decided to build a national resource where blind people could receive formal training because rehabilitation of the newly blinded had evolved significantly. In addition, the teaching of how to use a white cane to get about safely and efficiently had become specialized.

Divisions were encouraged to offer similar training on a local level to the elderly blind. Younger people and those needing more intensive specialized rehabilitation training were offered the opportunity to attend the A.V. Weir Centre on a residential basis. Another important dimension for the A.V. Weir Centre is that it allowed the CNIB to train rehabilitation specialists in applied skills and to formalize its personnel training in a range of specialties. International students were also accepted.

The A.V. Weir Centre concept, though, proved to be a hard sell to the operating divisions who had to help pay for it. The discussion went on for two years as the divisions argued they could offer the programs within their own facilities.

The divisions were right. The trend was moving toward community-based rehabilitation service, and in less than fifteen years the A.V. Weir Centre was used only occasionally for CNIB staff training.

With this phenomenal growth period, the picture seemed complete. Pearson Hall, on Beverley Street, had served the CNIB well for thirty-eight years, and if you were a blind or deaf-blind person of any age, or the parent of a blind child, the CNIB was virtually in your neighbourhood. The community also knew it. Whatever service was needed, whatever problem had to be solved, whatever issue had to be resolved, the

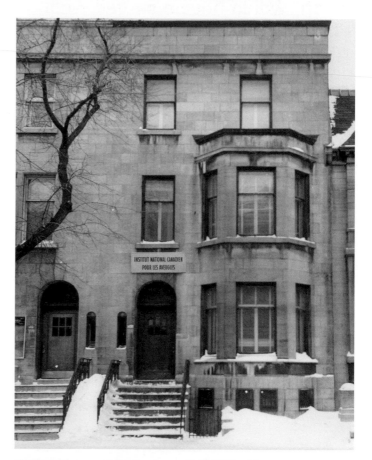

Ramsay House, 1459 Crescent Street, Montreal.

referral circle inevitably closed at the CNIB's front door.

Other than in Montreal, where there were two non-CNIB facilities, across Canada the CNIB was well on the way to fulfilling its founders' dreams as it delivered services to Canada's blind and visually impaired from coast to coast. The third coast, the far north, would not be served well until 1986 when a district office was established in Yellowknife;

much later, one opened in Whitehorse as well.

With firm roots in urban and rural Canada, the still relatively young institute had become a streamlined, successful national organization, cost-effective and well managed. Underpinning its success were the founders, staff members, and volunteers who had been on board since the beginning. But they were aging, and times were changing.

CHAPTER 10
Circling the Wagons

By 1960, with the exception of educational services and the two Montreal-based organizations, the CNIB had a solid hold on almost everything related to blindness in Canada.

Educational institutions, government departments and large employers relied upon or deferred to institute personnel for advice and guidance. This sphere of influence also extended to legislated provisions, and if you were a blind person in Canada, you had to show your CNIB registration card if you wanted access to reduced travel, cinema passes, or other concessions. For seventy years, CNIB internal policy had the same requirement to purchase white canes and other technical devices.

The CNIB had set up an elaborate network with agencies and programs in the United States and had negotiated formal agreements with them relating to library services, guide dog schools, distance learning, blindness prevention programs, and training in low vision services for staff. While the costs were not necessarily passed on to the client, the CNIB in several instances paid a minimal fee to purchase services from these organizations, which included the Hadley School for the Blind in Illinois. Referral to, and eligibility for, these services was screened and directed by CNIB staff either in Toronto or in the divisional offices to the extent that it was difficult, if not impossible, to get a guide dog unless the CNIB said you could have one.

Less formal, but equally effective, agreements existed in respect to fundraising; American agencies, with one notable exception, did not cross into Canada to raise funds, and neither did the CNIB raise funds in the U.S. The exception was an American-based church with legal status in Canada, which ignored the unwritten understanding and carried on elaborate fundraising campaigns for purposes that many believed questionable, such as library services and children's camps.

A common practice, which still occurs today, was for a rival blindness organization, or one purporting to be raising money to benefit the blind, to create confusion among donors by conducting a campaign ahead of the CNIB, so when a CNIB canvasser called to ask for a donation, the donor would think he had already given to the CNIB. In fact, his money had gone to another organization, which may or may not have been legitimate.

Blind people who needed a white cane or who wanted to buy special devices such as braille watches, games, craft supplies, and emerging technology were limited to dealing directly with the CNIB as these supplies were cataloged and sold at cost through the national and local offices. While it was possible to deal directly with the few suppliers that for the most part were international, it was just more convenient to deal directly with Blindcraft, as it was sometimes called.

Fewer than a dozen senior managers, all men and most of them blind, kept tight control on the levers of power. To be sure, a few women were also to be found at this level (but with noticeably less authority), including the recording secretary, the national eye service nurse, the national social services director, and a registrar. The war-blinded had their own designated after-care officer, but he reported to the managing director, with appropriate delegation, as did all others employed by the institute regardless of their position or location.

The National Council, made up of forty-six members, met only twice a year; a smaller Executive Committee functioned as the policy and governance body. Under the bylaws, members of the institute were eligible to attend the annual general meeting and vote, in person or by proxy. At the AGM, the corporate body would receive and approve the annual report, appoint auditors, and elect the new council, which had the power to then appoint officers. CNIB bylaws called for one-third of council members to be clients of the institute, that is, blind or visually impaired.

In each geographic division, the affairs were directed by boards of management. Although these boards were elected by various methods, they were, in fact, creatures of the National Council that established them by resolution and ratified the membership of each board annually. Within each province, the board of manage-

ment appointed advisory boards and committees with similar devolution of delegated authority with the ultimate authority retained by the council. Membership on all division boards continues to be ratified by the national board.

The military background of Managing Director Edwin Baker and others at a senior level had left a distinct imprint on the organizational culture and management style. Appointments of senior provincial staff were made in Toronto and rubber-stamped by local boards. Vacancies were filled by invitation, affording little opportunity for advancement for anyone wanting to move up within the organization. This approach was in no way intended to be disrespectful to staff and volunteers who were passed over, it was simply the way business was conducted.

The formal, militaristic management style of the CNIB could be seen every day at lunchtime in the Bayview cafeteria for an entire generation when Baker and his closest advisors, all men, sat at one table and in an established pecking order. While there was no written rule preventing women or others from joining them at the table, it just wasn't done; one would be part of this group by invitation only.

This autocratic management style was in marked contrast to other large national not-for-profit organizations that incorporated and operated along provincial or municipal lines and whose head offices functioned as an amalgam of loose-knit federations.

Another distinction that separated the CNIB from other disability organizations was the peculiar fact that blindness as a sensory loss was not regarded solely as a health issue, but rather was perceived more as a welfare or social issue. This accounts for the fact that throughout its history the CNIB retained cross-ministerial relations within governments at all three levels. Over time, this proved to be both an asset and a liability. The advantage was that there were more doors to knock on, but the disadvantage was that relationships were somewhat fragmented and spread out.

The governance and operating structure that had been in place since the founding of the CNIB had not changed very much across the decades. What was about to

change was the key players, and this upheaval had a resounding impact on the organization. From 1962 to 1969, beginning with the retirement of Baker himself, eight senior men and one key woman retired. Perhaps, like most of us, they had either considered themselves irreplaceable or couldn't bring themselves to believe that the day would actually come when they would retire, but for some reason, not much in the way of succession planning seems to have been done.

Three people — Lady Virginia Kemp (1954–1958), Ralph S. Misener (1958–1963), and His Honour Judge Frank G.J. McDonagh (1963–1965) — had served as president of National Council since Lewis Wood's retirement in 1954.

CHANGING TIMES

During this period, the CNIB had to weather not only a dramatic change in leadership after some forty years but also external forces affecting the organization. With the introduction of the Canada Assistance Plan in 1966, with its provisions that shifted federal/provincial relations and modified revenue sharing, public policies had been dramatically altered. The Canada Health Act brought similar adjustments, and these and other major initiatives by the federal government tweaked the balance of powers outlined in the British North America Act.

Although Quebec had not yet elected a separatist government, La Révolution tranquille was well under way. Mainstream education for disabled children was mandated, affirmative action programs were beginning to open more inclusive employment opportunities, and some three hundred young blind men and women were enrolled in post-secondary education.

The concept of normalization was paving the way for more inclusive lifestyles for the disabled of all ages, including people who were institutionalized or attending special residential schools.

Pan-disability groups, as they became known, began to emerge, driven largely but not exclusively by paraplegic young adults. Soon, these groups became vocal and effective pressure groups directing their complaints and requests toward governments and the line agencies that delivered services. Unlike blind, deaf-blind, and visually impaired people, other groups of disabled people had access to public health programs and rehabilitation facilities funded by universal medical care and operated, for the most part, by provincial governments. This was essentially the beginning of a curious practice of government funding the very pressure and lobby groups that organized protests directed back against the hand that fed them.

Much of this organized capacity attracted grants and was focused on public opinion and attitudinal shifts. Provocative and carefully crafted statements drew media attention that in turn began to shape and mould heightened public knowledge and awareness. Streams of diverse public funding empowered the consumer-owned and -driven organizations to draw attention to their causes, which in turn led them to demand a seat at the table where decisions were made and power was wielded. A satisfactory response to this request, however, was to prove elusive as boardroom doors were not easily pried open, and some, including the CNIB's, remained firmly closed.

A few blind individuals chose to align themselves with this generic self-help movement. Most were members of the Canadian Council of the Blind, as their collective consumer voice. By the mid-1970s, at least seven provinces had new organizations of blind and visually impaired people. In every case, what these groups lacked in membership they made up in volume — they were extremely vocal, often loud in their criticisms, and sometimes even aggressive in the Sol Olinsky school of social change that had swept North America and elsewhere.

The CNIB, as the natural leader for blindness rehabilitation, employment, library, recreation, and advocacy services, found itself a target at the centre of this new development, having neither encouraged nor assisted in founding the movement.

THE ROYAL COMMISSION

Folklore surrounding the wagon trains that marked the great western migration in America describes how, at the day's end, the wagons were drawn into a tight circle as a means of protecting the settlers from enemies that often were more imagined than real. Not unlike those early pioneers, the CNIB wagons were circled against this phenomenon, much as they had done in the 1930s.

Royal commissions come from our British heritage. Parliament passed an Inquiries Act in 1868, a similar act was passed in 1880, and then, in 1912 the two acts were combined into the Inquiries Act in use today. Except for the title chosen by whoever drafts the proclamation, royal commissions and commissions of inquiry are essentially the same thing.

In 1931 a Royal Commission was held "to inquire into all matters appertaining to the welfare of blind people within the provinces of Manitoba and Saskatchewan." This was the only time in its history the CNIB ever underwent such close scrutiny. From Confederation to the present day, about 450 official inquiries have been held, some royal commissions and some not. Judicial in nature, thorough, and an expensive charge on the public purse, some have done excellent work, bringing in far-sighted, workable recommendations and changing the country for the better. Others have been costly fiascoes. Many were called to deflect attention from a political hot potato, allowing the government of the day to say the matter "is under investigation," knowing that when the heat's off the report will benignly gather dust. On the plus side, however, these inquiries often provide vital material for long-range policy decisions and are valuable as vehicles for consciousness-raising as they bring issues out into the open for examination and discussion.

From the time of its establishment in 1919, the Central Western division for Manitoba and Saskatchewan had been struggling at the senior management level with issues related to distribution of CNIB funds, pensions for blind people, work placements, leadership, and whether or not the CNIB's national office was too involved in the running of the division, even to the point of using coercion.

The growing concerns eventually reached into the legislatures of both provinces at the highest level when the two premiers of the day, J.T.M. Anderson of Saskatchewan and R.A. Hoey, acting premier of Manitoba, arranged for a Royal Commission to look into the problems facing the blind in the two provinces.

An American, Olin H. Burritt, principal of the Pennsylvania Institute for the Blind, was appointed commissioner of the inquiry. His previous experience included undertaking a similar mission for the state of Pennsylvania a few years previous. Baker's words were measured on learning of the appointment. On April 22, 1930, he wrote to Major E. Flexman, Manitoba division superintendent in Winnipeg: "Mr. Burritt is an elderly gentleman who has spent all his adult life running a school for the blind. His knowledge of work for adult blind may be extensive but I am not so sure that he is fully equipped with up-to-date methods."

Six areas were identified for inquiry by the commission: prevention of blindness, conservation of vision, education and subsequent employment of the youthful blind, training and employment of the adult blind, teaching adult blind in their homes, and relief for the aged and infirm blind.

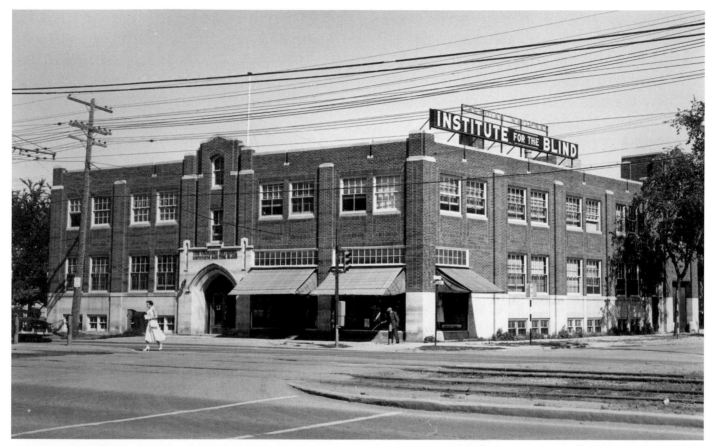

Central Western division headquarters at 1031 Portage Avenue, Winnipeg.

Allegations for the commission to investigate directed against the CNIB were blunt. "Failed in its trust" and "dominated by National Office" were expressed publicly. It would appear that the unrest was limited to Winnipeg and was galvanized on three major issues: the workshop, pensions, and education of blind students.

In 1930, forty-six blind people were employed in the workshops: thirty manufacturing brooms, ten in basketry, and six women sewing white ware goods (items like aprons and nurses' uniforms). The truth about sheltered workshop programs, in every disability field and in all countries then and now, is that there exists a dichotomy between paying sub-minimum wages to workers of varying abilities and subsidizing an operation that is often unprofitable. It was for those reasons that the CNIB closed its Halifax shop early on and transferred many of the workers to Toronto. The Winnipeg shop was started in 1921 with a $6,000 grant, which was never repaid, from the national office. The result was that by 1930 there were more workers than jobs, with growing demands and no options on the open market, especially as the country was on the brink of a massive economic depression that struck hard and long in Western Canada.

Blind workers in England had pressed for pension legislation as early as 1893, and by 1920 they had succeeded. Philip Layton, an Englishman who had immigrated to Canada, knew firsthand that a concerted effort would be required if the British experience were to succeed in Canada, and to that end he convened the first conference of blind Canadians in Montreal in September 1926. He then set out at his own expense to travel the country promoting the Canadian Federation of the Blind and to organize pressure groups for a blind pension. Thus, in 1930, in Winnipeg, four groups joined to form the United Blind Pension Committee of Manitoba. Lux In Tenebris, the CFOB, the CNIB, and Women's Auxiliary sent representatives. Their combined concerns, directed at both levels of government, added to the growing outcry among blind people in the run-up to the commission.

The idea of establishing a residential school for the blind in Western Canada was also being looked at. The Ontario School for the Blind, founded in 1872, had accepted five blind students prior to 1906, four from Manitoba and one from the Northwest Territory (which was Saskatchewan and Alberta by 1905). From 1906 to 1930, the three provinces were sending an average of thirty students each year. Train fare was $50 for children under twelve and $75 over twelve. Tuition of $300 for each student was charged to the provinces.

The commission explored several options for a residential school closer to home. Saskatoon was considered as a potential site to serve the three Western provinces, or Winnipeg for just Manitoba and Saskatchewan. The cost of building a residential program was estimated to be $250,000. Using schools in the United States was also considered, including the School for the Blind in Bathgate, North Dakota, south of Manitoba, which had thirty-five students.

After visiting the schools in Canada and consulting the Dominion Bureau of Statistics (the forerunner of Statistics Canada), Commission Chair Burritt concluded that there were at most fifty potential blind students. Price would also be a factor given that average costs ranged from $550 per student on a subsidized basis at the MAB school to $800 per student in Brantford and Bathgate. At $800 a head, Brantford was a bargain for the Prairie provinces, even though the children had far to travel and were away from their homes for ten months of the year, including over Christmas. It was recognized that Brantford and Montreal, which both accepted blind students from the West, had well-qualified, experienced teachers. The weight of this data precluded any serious view that a residential school would ever be constructed, but the issue never really died away as long as blind students were displaced from their families for as long as twelve years and sent either east to Ontario or west to Vancouver. Many of the children grew up as outsiders in their own families, not knowing their brothers or sisters.

The commission sat for sixteen days in the summer of 1930, listening to testimony from groups and individuals. In October, Burritt conducted a three-day site visit at the CNIB in Toronto, touring the workshops and attending a council meeting.

In March 1931, Burritt presented a lengthy and detailed formal report to both legislatures, which took the report seriously enough to appoint select committees to study it and make recommendations on its content. The report lavished praise on the CNIB. Burritt admired both Baker and Weir for their abilities, and in his summation of the CNIB's programs he wrote, "The United States has much to learn from the CNIB."

Much of the report dealt with the issue of poverty among blind people. To address the problem, a proposed solution based on the relief laws in existence in several states was put forward. The provisions for eligibility reflected the public attitudes of the day toward blind people. Ineligible in some jurisdictions were "Beggars and people with vicious habits." Blind people who married each other after the legislation was enacted were, in some cases, ineligible for more than one pension or, at best, one and a half times the allowance. The underlying intent was clear: to provide a better pension would be to encourage inter-marriage among the blind.

However, there may be another explanation for this, says social policy historian Shirley Tillotson:

> All pensions, whether old age, mothers', or work-men's compensations, were discontinued or halved for women when they married. So a female old age pensioner who married lost half her pension, and a woman who had been collecting a pension as the widow of a workman killed on the job would lose all of it if she remarried.

So while there was certainly a eugenicists' bias against people with disabilities, pension regulations in the period from 1920 to 1960 make me think that the bias was actually against treating married women as if they had an entitlement to equal income.

Colonel Baker, who was married to a sighted woman, opposed blind people marrying each other, describing the marriage as like a "house without windows." Gloria Sewell, a CNIB rehabilitation teacher and district administrator who also worked with the Children's Aid Society in Manitoba, married a blind CNIB employee and describes the marriage, with its ups and downs and challenges like any other marriage, in her book, *House Without Windows*.

Relief laws for the blind were never adopted in Canada, which opted for a national pension program, as described earlier. The Manitoba government stopped short of building a residential school for the blind but through the Department of Education operated a day school in Winnipeg, which was housed at the CNIB building at Portage and Sherburn streets from 1931, when it opened, until 1945, when it moved to the Margaret Scott School. Shortly afterwards, the school was closed, and blind students from all three Western provinces were sent to the Brantford School.

The long-term impact of the Royal Commission's report is difficult to assess. However, one factor was clear. Blind people could and would have their voices heard on major issues that directly affected their quality of life. There would be no going back. Issues related to employment, welfare, and education fit squarely into the public domain and the elected legislators. But the reality nevertheless persisted, perhaps to the comfort and convenience of successive governments, that the CNIB continued to draw the anger and disillusionment of blind people until a time in Canadian public policy when a safety net was broadened to include the needs of blind citizens. Or did it?

As for Major Flexman, he continued to serve until the outbreak of the Second World War, when he left to oversee a munitions plant in Ontario.

CHAPTER 11
The Twelve-Year Decade

For forty-four years the CNIB had experienced slow, orderly growth in services, staff, and facilities; but from 1962 to 1974, a short stretch of twelve years, events would redraw the organizational map all the way to the millennium. Some of this change was anticipated, but most was not.

This was not yet the era of consultants, massive reports, and cyclical strategic plans that required organizational effort on a "bottom-up" model. National management meetings were not held very often, semi-annually at best. The workshop and commercial catering activities were sizeable and in many ways operated almost independently of the service side.

The division versus national office tug-of-war was always delicate, imposing constraints on divisional operating budgets as they were required to finance the national office. It can be assumed that many lively discussions, took place over this issue. Revenue-sharing practices varied over time with different, often multiple formulae, including how to distribute bequest income. No fewer than nine parallel accounting departments were needed to track annual income and expenditures. Also, the CNIB had opted to become a part of, and in numerous places a charter member of, community appeals and what would eventually become United Ways or Centre Aides, severely restricting their in-house fundraising capacity. Provincial governments' granting mechanisms had moved from annual generic grants to more complex "purchase of service" agreements as they sought cost recovery from the federal government in areas such as vocational training. The federal government, in turn, offered sustaining grants to national organizations for both training and operations, All this required more accounting personnel, generated a massive paper flow, and demanded that organizations knock on many ministers' doors. As the source of their funds, these departments then expected input into what the organizations' agendas should be.

That, in turn, tended to drive the service to be offered; in other words, agencies began to develop

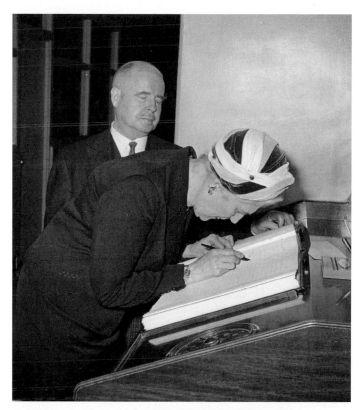

Judge Frank McDonagh, then vice-president of National Council, watches as Her Excellency Pauline Vanier, wife of Governor General Georges Vanier, signs the CNIB guest book, 1962.

services in response to needs that may or may not have really existed, in the chase for dollars from the public purse. This gradual, subtle shift had the further effect of raising the institute's reliance on external funding from United

Appeals and governments to 75 percent of its annual operating budget. Thirty years later this funding formula was completely reversed; by 2000, the CNIB was raising 80 percent of its revenue privately, with the government contributing only 20 percent.

Subsidies for workshops, catering, and residences contributed measurably to the bottom line, supporting administration costs of doing business. The one exception that stood out, as it had all along, was the national braille music and audio library that by now was serving many thousands of patrons from one central department at BakerWood. How to fund a rapidly expanding, high-demand program from internal sources sparked a debate that would not soon be resolved. By 1974, if you were blind and needed library or other materials for education, employment, or leisure, the CNIB national library was your only resource. For French readers, French braille was available from L'Institut Nazareth, with limited braille from the CNIB's Quebec division, but few audio books in French. There was also an impressive braille music collection in

Montreal. The doors to the public libraries, however, were firmly closed to sightless Canadians, as was the public purse that released funds for braille and special materials only to schools for the blind.

The public, if they thought about it at all, believed that the CNIB took care of all blind people from cradle to grave, and some probably thought it was part of a government ministry, at some level. Some CNIB staff groups, including administrative staff and CaterPlan workers, belonged to the collective bargaining units that had been certified in Saskatchewan, Manitoba, Ontario, Quebec, and later Newfoundland. "Tough love" in negotiations would change the climate within the organization. Strikes and walkouts occurred in Edmonton, Winnipeg, Toronto, and Montreal. Some were peaceful, others were much harsher, and the CNIB was now facing an unfriendly media when presenting its management position. Sophisticated public relations training in crisis management and media relations for top executives was still a few years away.

Blind people picketing on sidewalks outside CNIB buildings,

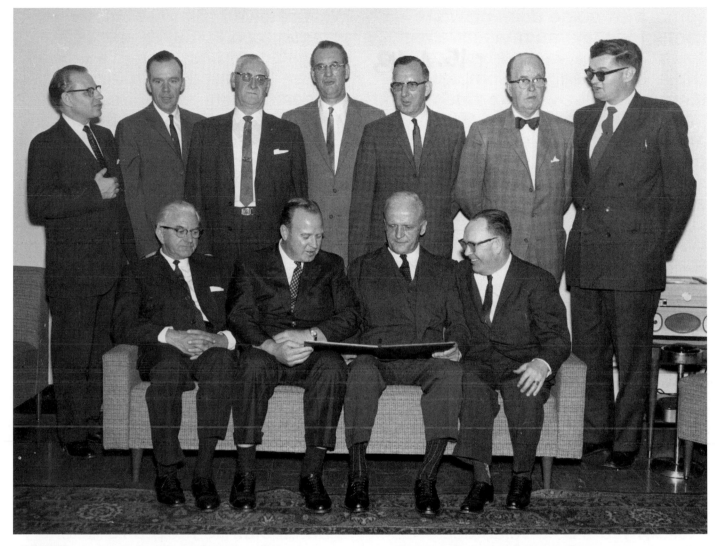

CNIB superintendents from across Canada gathered to congratulate Edwin Baker on his retirement, 1962. Back row (left to right): William Milton, Quebec; Ross Purse, Saskatchewan; A.W. Sparks, Ontario; S.J. Evans, Manitoba; Arthur Magill, managing director; M.C. Robinson, B.C.-Yukon; R.L. Storey, Manitoba. Seated (left to right): Frank Flinn, Maritimes; R.S. Misener, president; Edwin Baker, honorary president; S.D. Edmonson, Alberta.

some with guide dogs or white canes for maximum visual effect, might have invited comparison to those blind beggars from days long gone. But vocal, strident blind people waving placards at staff and passersby did nothing to support the CNIB's image as a professional, prestigious service organization with the best interests of its clients in mind.

This, then, was something of the climate at the CNIB in July 1962, when Baker handed over the managing director's position to Arthur (Art) Magill. Baker, who had insisted that CNIB staff retire at age sixty-five, had exempted himself from that policy and stayed on until he was sixty-nine. His son, John, later reflected that perhaps his father had stayed too long at the end. True or not, Baker had given the CNIB forty-six years of his life, beginning in 1916 and including the first six years as a volunteer.

Immediately after his retirement Baker was elected honorary president of National Council, and he and his secretary, Grace Worts, retained an office at BakerWood, partly to allow him to complete his international assignment as president of the World Council for the Welfare of the Blind. Worts, who was devoted to Baker, worked alongside him for many years and was an influential and dedicated support to him.

In 1983, as a tribute to the long and dedicated service she had given the organization, the CNIB established the CNIB Grace Worts Staff Service Award. This award is presented annually to an employee or former employee in recognition of a distinguished and valued career with demonstrated leadership and outstanding commitment to the advancement of services to blind and visually impaired Canadians.

ARTHUR MAGILL

Magill, who was born in Cobourg, Ontario, lost the sight in one eye in a crib accident when he was six months old. He moved to Regina as a child with his family, worked in construction from about the age of twelve, and then, in his mid-teens, moved back to Ontario. Sadly, he lost the sight in his other eye when an unthinking co-worker at the photofinishing shop where he was working fired a paper clip off a rubber band into his eye. Magill was sent to the School for the Blind in Brantford at the age of seventeen, did well, and was encouraged to stay in school. His family then moved to Michigan because there wasn't a high school in Ontario that would take him, and Magill went on to Michigan State University, where he earned a master's degree in business administration, with honours.

His career aspirations at this point, however, were thwarted; although he wanted to become a lawyer or professor, he was told that these career choices were not open to him because of his blindness.

Throughout this period of time in the 1930s, Baker was taking a quiet interest in Magill and even travelled several times to Michigan to visit him. Although he encouraged him to return to Canada to join the CNIB, Baker made sure young Magill with his business degree started at the bottom: his first job was slinging pop cases at the CNIB booth at Toronto's Royal Winter Agricultural Fair. Magill went on to become a district manager in Brantford and held various positions of increasing responsibility in the Ontario division, including serving as its director for ten years.

In her biography of Colonel Baker, Marjorie Wilkins Campbell wrote:

Colonel Baker's personal choice of a successor had been an open secret for months. He had long been grooming A.N. Magill as the second managing director of the CNIB, not in the belief or with the wish that Magill would follow him implicitly, but because he trusted the younger man to serve the needs of Canada's blind persons intelligently and with his own brand of dedication. To Magill and the new, younger group of personnel already coming on, he was willing to entrust the torch he had brought from St Dunstan's.

Interestingly, in an interview recorded in 1973, Magill stated that he felt he'd had no real training in preparation for assuming the top job. Be that as it may, he had been working for the CNIB at the management level for over twenty-five years, and it's difficult to see who else might have been promoted ahead of him, with two possible exceptions.

DAVID BAXTER LAWLEY

Born in Lancashire, England, in 1888, David Baxter Lawley was an interesting and capable man. He came to Canada in 1912 and lost his sight in 1913 through a dynamite explosion in the mine where he was employed.

Joining the CNIB staff in 1932, he organized boards and committees in Ontario and set up service to the blind on a district level. In 1936 he became the first supervisor of the Ontario Field Service Department and continued to develop the district program over the next ten years. In 1946 Lawley became national consultant of field services, and in 1947 he was loaned to the Trinidad and Tobago Association for more than a year to assist with establishment of services to the blind in the West Indies. Later, he served as acting superintendent of the Ontario divi-

sion, where he directed service programs to more than seven thousand blind Ontarians. He retired in 1956 and died in 1964.

In the same 1973 interview, Magill mused that Lawley "felt overlooked and unappreciated," and he went on to comment on Lawley's significant contribution.

WILLIAM E. MILTON

Born in Saskatchewan, William (Bill) E. Milton was sent at a young age to the school run by the Montreal Association for the Blind rather than the one in Brantford. In the 1930s, he and two other blind students attended a local high school before going on to university; they were among the first of a select group of fewer than ten blind students to be integrated into mainstream education. Milton was superintendent in two divisions: he was the first superintendent in Alberta from 1956 to 1958 when it was established as a separate division, and he was superintendent in Quebec from 1958 to 1965. On January 1, 1966, after suffering a heart attack, he took up his new position as national director, vocational guidance.

In 1979, he was appointed national consultant to senior management by Managing Director Ross Purse, who is effusive in his praise for Milton's contribution. Milton retired in 1982 and died soon after.

His wife, Elizabeth, deserves special mention for the time she and Grace Worts, former executive assistant to the managing director, spent in transferring CNIB files tracing the history of the CNIB to the National Archives in Ottawa for safekeeping. With help from others, they reviewed some fourteen hundred files and forwarded the entire collection to Ottawa, where it was cross-indexed by subject. Thanks to their efforts, the National Archives now holds forty-five boxes of historic documents that provide an invaluable treasury of information. The project took over seven thousand hours of volunteer time and took three and a half years to complete.

NEW DEVELOPMENTS

Claude Gauthier began his work with the CNIB by volunteering as a CNIB district board member. He also conducted fundraising campaigns for twelve years. His sight began to fail, and in 1960 he attended, along with four others, the first Adjustment to Blindness course in Toronto, which meant living in the CNIB's Clarkewood Residence on Bayview Avenue for a four-month stay away from home and family.

Merv Carlton, a visually impaired Hong Kong veteran, arrived from Vancouver in September to teach students how to get about safely using a white cane. As canes became popular tools for safe, independent travel, it was realized that proper instruction was needed in how to use them.

Before Carlton arrived, Earl Green, a blinded veteran of the First World War, accompanied by his guide dog, travelled wherever he was needed in Canada to teach mobility.

Gauthier recalled that when Baker retired, Gauthier was seventh in a line of moves in Ontario from a domino effect. Alf Sparks replaced Magill in Ontario, four others moved to new assignments in the division, and Gauthier went to Ottawa assistant district administrator. In 1964, he was moved to Sudbury to replace Leslie Y. Jones, who, along with his driver, Ray Swarbrick, was tragically killed in a collision with a truck near Englehart, Ontario. The two had been driving to Virginiatown, on the Quebec border, to speak to a Lions Club. A second passenger, Jack Clemmons, survived.

A second tragedy occurred three years later in Sydney, Nova Scotia, when two field secretaries, George Wood and Emery Leblanc (who was training with Wood), drowned on a fishing trip when their eight-foot vessel overturned off Cape Breton Island. Also drowned was Wood's son, Robert. A second son, Richard, the only survivor, swam for six hours to get help.

Two fatal accidents and the loss of five lives within such a short time was an anomaly for the CNIB. For more than eighty years, CNIB staff and volunteers have travelled millions of kilometres in a vast country in all road and weather conditions, when staff were often working fourteen-hour days, seven days a week.

Gauthier's district encompassed northeast Ontario stretching to James Bay, more than twenty thousand square miles. He was the sole representative and employed one home teacher. That scope was typical of many other districts throughout Canada and in the north.

Change in leadership went beyond Ontario. Ross Purse had left Regina in 1961 to replace the retiring Captain M.C. Robinson of the B.C.-Yukon division. Stan Evans, who retired in 1966 from Manitoba, was replaced by Robert Storey, who moved with his family from St. John's.

In the Maritime division, Frank Flinn, whose father had been injured in the 1917 Halifax Explosion, had been recruited in 1934. Flinn, who was sighted, retired in 1969, adding to the list of retirees during the decade. He was succeeded by Ron Hill, who served until 1973. Hill had worked with Flinn since 1938 and had been instrumental in opening offices in Saint John, New Brunswick, in 1939, in Moncton, New Brunswick, in 1948, and in Charlottetown, Prince Edward Island, in 1949.

The Sydney, Nova Scotia, office opened in 1943. By 1956, five more offices had been opened in Bathurst, Edmonston, and

Fredericton in New Brunswick. Yarmouth and Truro, in Nova Scotia, were also added.

These new men were now Magill's management team. Bruce Belanger had taken on CaterPlan, and in 1964 Douglass Johnston became general manager, replacing Art Weir.

Johnston joined the staff in 1958 as assistant business manager in the Ontario division. Previously employed by leading Canadian food and manufacturing firms, he brought to the CNIB a wide experience in accounting, purchasing, marketing, general administration, and expansion planning. He also, apparently, brought along his ambitions.

Ralph Misener, a shipping magnate, served as president from 1958 to 1963, and during his term many of the new buildings were constructed. Although he resigned from the CNIB's top volunteer post because of the pressures of business, Misener continued to take an interest in CNIB affairs. He was succeeded by His Honour Judge Frank G.J. McDonagh, who oversaw the changing of the guard with the appointments of the new senior level managers. McDonagh,

who with Baker and Lewis Wood had assisted in the development of the CNIB in its early days, was elected to National Council in 1945. He also served as vice-president and honorary treasurer for some years and died in 1974.

POWER STRUGGLE

In 1950, George Thompson, who with his brother, Gordon, had incorporated Acadia Bus Lines, joined the Maritime division board at Flinn's encouragement. In 1938, in response to a request from Flinn for reduced bus fares for blind people, Acadia had granted the first such concession in Canada for inter-city bus travel.

Gordon was a quiet, modest man who took on the day-to-day operational tasks of running the bus line. In sharp contrast, George, the external voice who drove the business, hid the kind, thoughtful aspect of his personality under an aggressive, forceful manner. In 1966, he was elected national chair and served for seven years.

Magill's task was to carry on where Baker had left off — not an easy or enviable role. His calm personality and measured, quiet manner, in contrast to that of the assertive Baker, might have fooled some, including, perhaps, George Thompson and CNIB General Manager Douglass Johnston.

Magill was the third blind man to occupy the CNIB's most senior office, after Charles Holmes and Baker. The CNIB's bylaws mandate that the president and CEO must be a client, in other words blind or visually impaired. This became a serious issue.

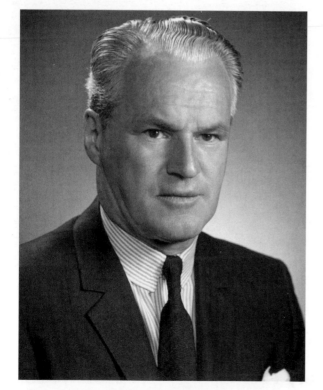

George Thompson.

Johnston, who was viewed as crafty and shrewd, wanted increasingly more decision-making power for himself. Among some serving on the council, Johnston was tacitly if not overtly encouraged. The somewhat passive Magill stood by, but after a time he decided that he, not Johnston, would be in sole charge.

George Thompson sided with Johnston, leading to a feud that divided the council and sparked a two-year power struggle. Few in the institute knew fully what was going on, and those who did were reluctant to talk about it, but lawyer John Magill, Art's son, spoke about the incident in an April 2003 interview recorded in Toronto.

Saying that his father was especially passionate about two causes in particular — access to higher education for blind youth and changing the paternalistic system of sighted people making decisions that affected the lives of blind people — John Magill said he did not know the details of the conflict, but he was aware of the effect it had on his father.

It was the only time in my memory that my

father was animated in his tone and he was very ... I never heard him raise his voice ever ... but he was more agitated and concerned about this than anything I can recall.

It was also difficult for my mother and father because the Johnstons lived not far from our house, they travelled to and from work together, attended functions together, and although certainly not close friends, they were well acquainted. Somehow, the two of them represented completely different sides on that issue.

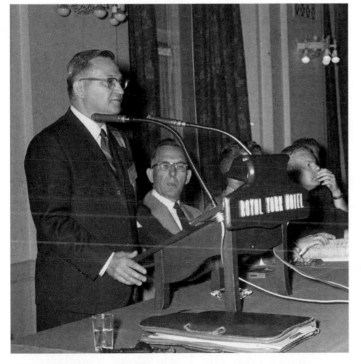

Douglass Johnston addresses a group at the Royal York Hotel, Toronto, while Arthur Magill looks on.

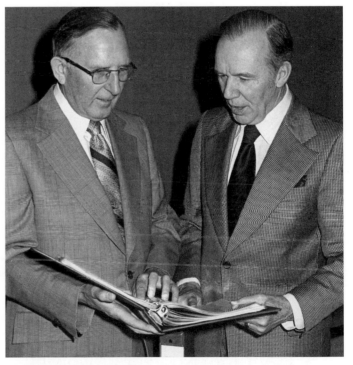

Arthur Magill, national consultant (left) with his successor, Managing Director Ross Purse, 1974.

In the end, Johnston was dismissed, and Thompson handed over the chairmanship of the council to George Beck in 1973, believing this to be in the organization's best interest.

The Magill-Johnston conflict had far more significance than simply a power struggle between two men at a senior level. The matter clearly demonstrated that a blind person could exercise legitimate authority in directing any operation, regardless of size and scope. Had Magill capitulated, an aura of defeat and discouragement for blind people in Canada and elsewhere would have been created. The attitude that blind people are limited to being senior managers sometimes exists in the minds of sighted trustees, so it is not surprising that most agencies for the blind in developed countries have been directed by sighted individuals. Clearly not so at the CNIB. Baker saw to that, and so did Magill.

Magill remained on staff as a consultant for two years following his official retirement in 1973.

To honour Magill, the council established the Arthur Napier Magill Distinguished Service Award, given annually to a volunteer who has made an outstanding contribution to the prevention of blindness or amelioration of conditions for blind Canadians. The award consists of a medal designed by Dora de Pedery-Hunt, a distinguished Canadian artist, and a scroll outlining the achievements of the award winner.

The first award, given at the CNIB's annual general meeting in May 1976, went to Marjorie McGuffin-Wood for her service to deaf-blind Canadians. McGuffin-Wood, herself deaf-blind, managed a home, raised three children, taught herself braille and how to type, and started *Dots and Taps*, a newsletter for the deaf-blind. The recipient of many awards, McGuffin-Wood was the CNIB's national consultant and personal worker for the deaf-blind until her retirement in 1973. She did much to raise awareness of deaf-blind issues.

The list of recipients is lengthy and impressive and includes, among others, Walter and Phyllis Gretzky.

Over time, the award acquired prestige and recognition as the institute's highest award for a volunteer; it became truly a credit to Magill's international service and his forty years as an employee and a fitting tribute to his memory.

ROSS PURSE

Ross Purse, who succeeded Magill as managing director in September 1973, lost most of his sight as a result of imprisonment in Hong Kong during the Second World War. After rehabilitation training at CNIB he began his career in the catering department. During the years that followed he worked in western Canada in several administrative positions and served as director of the Saskatchewan and B.C.-Yukon divisions. In 1969 he became divisional director of Ontario. Described as an approachable man, Purse was the first managing director since Charles Holmes to come from outside Ontario so he was expected to bring a fresh view to the front office.

Purse, who knew the organization well from the grass roots up, knew that troubled waters lay ahead. And the most turbulent of those waters were lapping the shores of the St. Lawrence River.

THE QUEBEC MELTDOWN

Geographic divisions had been up and running in the Maritimes and western Canada within three years of the institute's founding in 1918. But co-founders Lewis Wood and Edwin Baker believed that to be truly national, the CNIB would need a permanent presence in the province of Quebec, something that would not be achieved until 1931.

Baker's son, the late John R. Baker, who served as national chair from 1983 to 1987, affirmed that his father was determined to have Quebec become part of the national structure despite strong opposition from within the province.

In the 1920s, Quebec already had several organizations such as schools and workshops, most of them in Montreal, that served the blind. In 1861, L'Institut Nazareth was created, and in 1869, the MacKay Institute for Deaf-Mutes and Blind was founded by Joseph and Edward MacKay, bachelor brothers from Scotland who had made millions from their dry goods company on McGill Street.

Philip Layton, described as a high-energy visionary and an effective fundraiser, had arrived in Canada from England as a qualified piano tuner and accomplished organist, having been recruited by a Montreal church. When he arrived, the church elders realized he was blind and refused to hire him.

Undaunted, in 1909 Layton and a fellow blind piano tuner named Charles Lindsey founded the Montreal Association for the Blind, an English-speaking blindness organization, because they felt that anglophone blind people in Quebec did not have access to the same rehabilitation and education services as francophones. Following the MAB's founding, several French-only associations and workshop programs also sprang up.

Around 1912, the MAB acquired 5.2 hectares of land some distance west of the downtown core, in what is now Westmount. Recently, two small parcels of this land were sold, and with these funds, the MAB continues to operate a school, residence, and service centre offering a range of technical and rehabilitation programs.

In 1926, Layton obtained a federal charter forming the Canadian Federation of the Blind. This was intended to become Canada's first national consumer-driven advocacy group, and Layton travelled across the country to promote it and form provincial chapters.

The CFOB set up its headquarters in Regina, Saskatchewan, and with a national publication and fundraising arm, it was not only in serious competition with the emerging CNIB but was also a thorn in Baker's side. At times, the confrontations became bitter, with struggles for government approval and turf wars over fundraising among the various areas of the public.

Eventually, the CFOB fragmented into autonomous provincial structures, and it was formally dissolved in Saskatchewan in 1981. In other provinces, with the exception of the schools for the blind, the CNIB had been able to amalgamate blindness organizations into its fold. French-speaking Quebec, however, was different and proved difficult to negotiate with.

Although Baker and Wood made numerous representations and approaches to Quebec-based organizations throughout the 1920s, they met with little success. The argument they kept hearing was that the presence of yet another organization for the blind would be a duplication of existing ones, and the French organizations were proving resistant.

By 1930, Baker had obtained the support of the Grey Nuns, one or two associations, and a workshop. He also received support from the Council of Social Organizations and, significantly, Sir Charles Lindsey, and thus, despite the active opposition of Philip Layton and the MAB, a CNIB division was formed in Quebec in 1931.

Baker brought in Dr. John MacDonald from Halifax as the division's first superintendent. With its active and aggressive registration of French-speaking blind people, the Quebec division grew rapidly. By the 1950s, the CNIB had established sixteen district offices and advisory boards, along with a large residence in Quebec City with two workshops. The catering program employed over four hundred people with annual sales eventually reaching $15 million.

The CNIB joined the Red Feather appeal, a precursor to Centraide, and in the early days, it actually cooperated with the MAB in fundraising. Eventually, however, the MAB decided to strike out on its own and retain its independence.

From a retrospective point of view, for the first forty years the Quebec division's structure and service model replicated what existed in Ontario and elsewhere. In Quebec, the CNIB served a far larger number of blind people, mostly French speakers, than did the MAB. The services were also provincial and federal in scope with direct links to federal government programs for blind veterans, travel, and other concessions and tax credits.

And then suddenly in 1983, fifty-two years after its inception, the Quebec division suffered a dramatic and historic meltdown. Labour unrest and ruptured collective agreements, major shifts in provincial government policies, an eroded fundraising base, abandonment of membership in United Appeals, and well-orchestrated vocal consumer groups combined to provide insurmountable obstacles. To this mix was added increasing reliance for significant financial support from the CNIB's National Consolidated Fund. The Quebec division board struggled in vain to retain a viable operation.

The French language library, established in 1962 with a strong braille music component, had been relocated to Toronto amid huge opposition from blindness organizations, government, the media, and the public. Viewed through the lens of legislative requirements of the day, including the controversial French language requirements laid down in Bill 101, and given the public mood, the move was seen as a linguistic and cultural affront.

The library's French audio collection was eventually returned to Montreal from Toronto. In 1981, recognizing that the CNIB national library did not have the capacity nor the resources to produce French braille materials with the efficiency of the well-established transcription services in Quebec, the CNIB's National Council accepted a management recommendation to donate its French braille collection to Les Instituts Nazareth et Louis Braille on condition that all blind readers across Canada would be able to access the material.

How, then, did a healthy division with more than six hundred employees, an active and committed volunteer corps, sixteen service centres, a residence, a service centre in downtown Montreal, two workshops, and a French recording program for audio books and magazines serving twelve thousand clients dissolve into a division of a dozen staff offering limited service programs out of a rented office in Montreal in less than five years? How could the division's budget have shrunk from a gross operation of $15 million per year to $1 million by 1983?

Possible explanations depend on your point of view and whether you are looking at the issue from within the CNIB or from outside the organization as a client, policy maker, casual observer, or amateur historian.

Following La Révolution tranquille and the election of René Levesque's separatist government in 1976, the establishment of three para-public rehabilitation centres to serve blind people was mandated. The Centre Louis Hébert in Quebec City (located in the former CNIB residence and service centre) and the INLB in Montreal would serve French-speaking clients, and the MAB in Montreal would serve the anglophone population.

A media report cited in Susanne Commend's book *Les Instituts Nazareth et Louis-Braille, 1861–2001: Une Histoire de Coeur et de Vision* on the history of the INLB states that the CNIB turned down an offer to become a special technology centre. Be that as it may, clearly the CNIB fell outside the government's scope of programs, funding, and policies.

For some reason, the three designated centres were initially restricted from serving blind people over the age of twenty-one. This restriction was later amended to people over the age of thirty-five, and only much later, in 1992, was the restriction lifted so blind people of all ages could be helped. Services in rural and remote areas were and are provided on a multi-disciplinary model through the local health centres.

In the 1980s and 1990s, the CNIB in Quebec attempted to serve those people not eligible for services from the government-funded centres but was unsuccessful. The blindness prevention programs, including a mobile eye care unit, were eventually discontinued, leaving registration and referral as the main services. A comprehensive

technology program and quality French recording studios, later digitized, left a measure of credibility.

Part of the issue was that after 1976, provincial funding could not, under the social legislation, be granted to a non-Quebec organization. Visions of funds leaving the province and heading to Toronto influenced the perceptions, if not the reality.

In response, in 1980 the CNIB's National Council registered the CNIB Quebec division under a separate provincial charter. L'Institut National des Aveugles du Quebec remains on the books in Quebec City, but its existence never resulted in a single provincial contribution. The employment program did receive a large subsidy through the federal/provincial funding formula, but the program was transferred to a consumer group due solely to anti-CNIB pressures with the Quebec government.

Could the outcomes have been different? Perhaps. It was certainly unfortunate that with central structure and control of the CNIB in Toronto, no one spoke French at the time and no one recognized or understood that the climate in Quebec was changing rapidly. This serious lack of intelligence and judgment stood for several years, and by the time it was recognized, it was too late.

However, a lesson may have been learned in time to respond to similar pressures and shifting priorities by the government of New Brunswick, as National Council moved rather quickly to form its tenth operating division. Much of what is recorded here was confirmed during a 2003 interview with Gerald Tremblay, a prominent Montreal lawyer, honorary life member of the CNIB, and former Quebec CNIB board chair.

A reflective Tremblay, who, with his predecessor chairs Susan Clark and Gerald St. Denis, presided over much of the meltdown, said it would have been "almost foreign" for the Quebec government of the day to have recognized or funded a national organization from Toronto.

Also in 2003, Dr. John Sims, executive director of the MAB from 1977 to 1986, confirmed not only the Tremblay observations but also the early history of the Baker-Layton era.

CHAPTER 12
THE RENAISSANCE YEARS

To suggest that the CNIB train had left the station with the appointment of Ross Purse as managing director in 1973 would be to understate the elements of change that occurred in the ensuing decade.

Only twice in the institute's history of nearly a century have both the president and board chair been blind or visually impaired. The unstated practice seemed to be that a healthier balance of powers would exist if the chair were sighted, because under the CNIB bylaws, the president must be a client. This arrangement may have been partly tradition and partly a hangover from the Magill-Johnson incident.

The first time two blind or visually impaired people held these two key positions occurred from 1973 to 1977, when George Beck was chair and Ross Purse was managing director. The second instance occurred about thirty years later, when Frances Cutler of Ottawa was the chair from 2000 to 2003. During her time, Euclid Herie stepped down as president and was replaced by James Sanders. This system of having a sighted chair lead the governing boards was copied in the divisions, with few exceptions, until the closing years of the twentieth century.

Beck and Purse had both been left visually impaired as a result of horrific war injuries. Born and educated in Toronto at Crescent School and then at Upper Canada College, Beck was a commissioned officer on loan to the British Army as a CanLoan officer when he was wounded in Italy in 1944. He had been left for dead after a fierce battle, propped up against an old wall with nothing but a water canteen to sustain him, in the belief that his wounds would soon claim his remaining hours of life. Discovered by medics some time later, he was transferred back to England where he underwent extensive rehabilitation (but not at St Dunstan's).

After the war, he joined the bond firm of Andras, Bartlett, Cayley Ltd. as a junior and remained to become president of the company. His strong family values might have made Norman Rockwell envious. Tall, affable, and ebullient, Beck never wavered in his unshakeable trust in the work of the CNIB. No two men could have differed more in nature and leadership style than did Beck and his predecessor, George Thompson. This change in organizational chemistry came not a minute too soon as the train chugged ever forward to an unknown destination.

Purse was returned to Canada shortly after the cataclysmic explosion of the atomic bombs over Japan that ended the Second World War. At that time Purse, with many other Canadians, was working as slave labour in Japanese mines, and he is unequivocal in his belief that "had it not been for the atomic bomb, none of us would have survived another winter." Emaciated and near death when he was released, Purse would suffer chronic health problems as a consequence of his four years as a prisoner of war in Hong Kong and Japan.

Unlike his predecessor, Art Magill, who had worked in only one division (Ontario), Purse was very much a "field" man in that he moved around and worked in four divisions. After his post-war rehabilitation, Purse joined the CNIB in

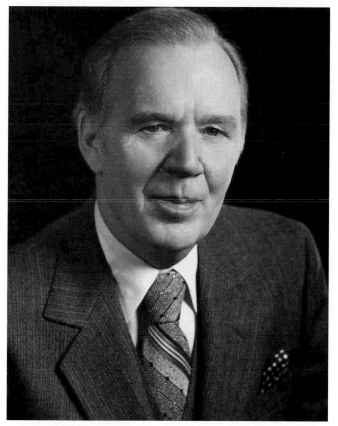

Ross Purse.

then moved on to senior positions in British Columbia and Ontario in a progressive career path that almost organically brought him to the head of the organization.

Twenty years at a senior management level not only prepared Purse for his new duties as managing director but also gave him a real ability to take the pulse of the organization and the services it provided. Purse also brought to the position a realistic sense of the external environment and an uncanny ability to size up shifts in public policy. He had no doubt that the CNIB needed to work harder in reaching its external audiences, and within the CNIB, he was passionate about training and education for employees and blind youth.

The dapper Purse projected a serious corporate image while bringing an underlying sensitivity and good humour to his role. His war experiences had taught him the importance of careful planning, patience, and attention to detail. In later life, he prided himself on having spotted early on the potential in his three successors: Robert Mercer, Euclid Herie, and James Sanders.

Manitoba in the canteen program where he spent three months sweeping floors and stocking shelves. From there, he entered the field service and in 1955 moved to Regina to direct the provincial services as part of the Central Western division.

In 1961 he became the first superintendent in Saskatchewan when that province was established as a separate division. Purse

Until 1970 it was a well-established practice at the CNIB to promote from within whenever possible. In the early years of his appointment, Purse changed this by reaching outside the organization to recruit senior management. Robert Mercer and Euclid Herie, who went on to become CNIB presidents, and Françoise Hébert, director of CNIB library services, were all brought into the organization this way. It should be noted, however, that for many years the organization has had a written policy that when candidates with equal qualifications are being considered for a job, preference will be given to the person who is blind or visually impaired.

By 1977 the CNIB National Library (still a department and not yet a division) and virtually all eight geographic divisions were under new management, and the look of the CNIB was dramatically altered. For one thing, a woman line manager, Françoise Hébert, had joined the table for the first time.

BOOST

In 1973, blind people held an important meeting at the St. Lawrence Hall in Toronto. Claude Gauthier and Ontario Manager Joe Caruk were in attendance to observe the founding of BOOST (Blind Organization of Ontario with Self Help Tactics). For the next ten years and beyond, this group would pressure and antagonize the CNIB relentlessly. Their attacks came in many forms, reminiscent of the Sol Olinsky school of protest that included locked-arm protests and a vigorous media campaign urging the CNIB to unlock its boardroom door to have open meetings and let them be board members.

In expressing their concerns, BOOST said the CNIB was a closed, secretive, paternalistic organization with a monopoly on services to the blind. BOOST claimed that blind people had no say in policy formation, an assertion which was at best unfair and at worst untrue. The CNIB was unmoved.

A 1980 BOOST report entitled "Developing Alternative Service Models" (also known as the DASAM report) included recommendations that in effect would have seen the CNIB, with its national reach, dismantled and replaced by provincial agencies along the lines of the U.S. state commissions for the blind. The report attracted mild media interest, but nothing came of it.

BRAM

In other provinces, groups were formed to champion similar issues. The difference in Ontario was that the target was easily accessible, right in the heart of Toronto, with the CNIB's national and provincial affairs offices located conveniently in one building.

In the Maritimes, six angry young blind students, who found themselves educationally disadvantaged compared to sighted students, formed BRAM (Blind Rights Action Movement). In response to their criticism, in 1972 the four Atlantic provinces commissioned David R. Lowry, assistant professor of law at Dalhousie University, to undertake an examination of the law relating to the blind in Canada, with particular reference to Nova Scotia. The Lowry report featured twenty-three recommendations, including that the CNIB should investigate impartially the charges of paternalism levelled by many against the personnel of the CNIB, that the province of Nova Scotia

should enact legislation which would facilitate compulsory attendance of blind children at a suitable educational establishment, that the school admissions system at the Halifax School for the Blind was inappropriate and inadequate, and that whenever possible, only properly trained teachers should be allowed to teach the blind. The report also stated: "The Halifax School for the Blind is inadequate and emphasis must be placed on the integration of the visual handicapped into the public school system. Only the small percentage of *totally* blind students should remain at the Halifax School for the Blind."

BRAM also set up a workshop, independent of the CNIB, to provide employment for blind people and to serve as a training ground for those seeking employment outside the workshop. The CNIB did, however, provide office support, and two of the BRAM pioneers, Robert Mercer and Chris Stark, became CNIB employees.

By the 1970s the CNIB had in place an active and effective public relations program, led by Paul O'Neill, national director. A quiet, gentle person, O'Neill had solid experience in internal communications, media relations, and special event planning. With an M.A., O'Neill began his career in the Ontario division, but by 1970 he had extensive experience of the organization at the national level. It was he who created the popular CNIB agenda book, still produced annually as a planned giving tool. O'Neill also served as an editor of the client newsletter, *National News of the Blind*, which was published from 1946 to 1981.

In the early 1980s, O'Neill and PR staff in other divisions were forced to respond to an unrelenting assault from groups of vocal blind people. The media were readily drawn in, often proving unsympathetic to CNIB viewpoints, and governments were forced to sit up and take note.

THE "UNMET NEEDS" STUDY

Purse, from his viewpoint in the corner office, knew all this, and he also knew another important fact: the federal government had decided to review its sustaining grant program for not-for-profit and charitable national organizations.

Purse approached a somewhat reluctant CNIB National Council and urged that a comprehensive, national internal review be undertaken. Commissioned in September 1974 by the National Council of the CNIB in co-operation with the federal Department of National Health and Welfare, Welfare Grants Directorate, an ambitious study to explore the unmet needs of blind Canadians was launched. The $90,000 cost of the study was shared between the CNIB and the government.

At the suggestion of Louise Cowan, the CNIB's coordinating consultant of social services and rehabilitation teaching, Cyril Greenland was chosen as project director of the "Unmet Needs" study.

Greenland, a graduate of the London School of Economics and a social worker, had been retained in 1958 by the Ontario government as a consultant to its mental health program. Greenland spent a year at the Whitby Mental Health Institute studying the organization's personnel and programs. There, he made the startling discovery that some sixty blind adults, none of whom was registered with or known to the CNIB, were hidden among the patient population. This was the largest single client group outside a school for the blind that the CNIB had ever encountered.

Cowan worked with Greenland to register these individuals and provide services to them. They were provided with watches and talking books, and in some cases, the people were re-housed independently in the community or moved to the CNIB's Clarkewood residence.

By 1974 Greenland had become well known as a social activist (with a national reputation for his work on child abuse) and as an expert on the history of psychiatry in Canada. He was a member of the faculty of the School of Social Work at Hamilton's McMaster University.

So with Cowan as chairperson, a national steering committee was established consisting of fourteen mainly blind representatives from diverse backgrounds, regions of Canada, ages, and work experience. Provincial groups were put in place, and for the next two years Greenland and Cowan shuttled back and forth across the country to consult, to chair public meet-ings, and to receive written sub-missions. Several thousand blind, visually impaired, and deaf-blind people took part in the process.

The study had four main objectives:

> To determine the current needs of visually handi-capped people; to deter-mine to what extent these needs are being adequately met by exist-ing agencies and pro-grams; to suggest what, if any, organizational and administrative changes are required to improve existing programs or to develop new ones; and to collect information on the special unmet needs of people with multi-handicaps such as the deafblind, blind retarded [sic] and others.

In addition to these objectives, it was also anticipated that the CNIB administration would under-take an in-house study to deter-mine how its staff and resources were being deployed to meet existing needs. Unfortunately, these in-house studies were either not undertaken or not completed in time to be included in the final report. It was also agreed that each division would undertake a parallel study of its own operations, and this aspect, too, fell short. Only in Manitoba, under the leadership of David Garvie, was a fairly comprehensive study done. The Manitoba board took the Garvie report seriously, with positive outcomes.

On August 26, 1976, Cyril Greenland's report was published in four volumes in English, French, braille, and cassette under the title *Vision Canada*.

The report documented the charge that in an affluent society, the blind are the poorest of the poor. It listed some fifty-four recommendations, focusing on nine key areas: blindness and poverty, human rights, health needs and vision care, education, rehabilitation and employment, communications, orientation and mobility, volunteers and the voluntary agency, and organizational problems and solutions. The recommendations were not all aimed at the CNIB but included governments, health services, education authorities, ophthalmologists, and community organizations.

The report took an unbiased, warts-and-all look at the problems. In his conclusions, Greenland wrote:

> The younger generation, tending to view themselves first as people, prefer not to be identified with their disability. Consequently, they are impatient with CNIB and seek to be fully integrated into society. The older generation, comprising over half all the registered blind Canadians, have more immediate and practical concerns. Many of them are trapped not only by the loss of vision but also by loneliness, poverty, poor health and all the other ills associated with being old and in a young country. However, unlike blind youth, older people depend on CNIB to do things for them.

The extent of unmet needs, revealed by this study, presents a great challenge to all Canadians. It is obvious that no single agency, however well intentioned and resourceful, will be able to overcome the years of neglect, prejudice and intolerance which is the common experience of handicapped people in our society.

The shocking conclusion should have caused a national outrage. Fully one hundred years of work with the blind had elapsed, and nowhere, with the publication of this report, was the brass ring within reach of blind Canadians.

Some of the recommendations, such as that the name of the CNIB should be changed to Vision Canada, were revolutionary, and others, for example that travel concessions should be abandoned in favour of cost of blindness allowances, were startling.

Greenland urged Canadian Press, the national co-operative news gathering agency, to provide a weekly digest of news and public affairs on cassette, to be available through the mail or public libraries. He accused the Canadian Broadcasting Corporation of scarcely recognizing the existence of blind people and recommended special programs on prime time radio and television.

Other recommendations were just plain common sense, for example that consumers should be invited to serve on CNIB division boards.

Greenland was in some respects critical of the CNIB. "In endeavouring to care for all the needs of blind people, CNIB tends to promise more than it or any group could deliver," he said. He claimed this CNIB approach was a disservice instead of a service, letting communities off the hook and removing their social responsibilities for their blind citizens. To restore this obligation the CNIB should remove itself from as many direct services as possible and train personnel in government, education, and other outside organizations to provide the programs. "CNIB should become a major resource for research, development and training for all the helping professions," he wrote, "specifically for education, social welfare, public health, medicine, science and technology."

The report was presented to National Council in April 1976, and a sub-committee, chaired by Betty Osler, was set up to study it and report back to the board. In November, the sub-committee duly presented fourteen recommendations, the committee was thanked, and the report was tabled and then, apparently, left to languish and gather dust.

The report, easily the most exhaustive study that had been undertaken to that point in the organization's history, received a mixed reaction within the CNIB. Some said it wasn't scientific, others were eager to accept its recommendations. However, because the study had taken two years, some of its components had been or were about to be implemented anyway.

Greenland, who had immersed himself fully and tirelessly in the project, received lavish praise and thanks from Purse in a 2003 interview. Both men admired and respected each other.

The report also brought the issues of blindness and visual impairment to a new level of awareness among Canadians. To the ongoing credit of Greenland and Cowan, supported by Purse, the Vision Canada study influenced how blind Canadians would be served in the years to come, and in many respects it was a renaissance document.

DAVID STANLEY

Tim Sheeres, who would later become national chair, asked David C.H. Stanley to volunteer on the council finance committee. Stanley, a brilliant professional in the finance field, had an exceptional and analytical mind. A private, shy individual, he became the institute's seventh chair of the National Council in May 1976. He believed that the chair should rotate every three years and was determined he would serve for only a three-year term.

His time in office was busy. During his tenure the CNIB entered the modern technology era with the conversion of library materials into a new audio format, launched the first capital campaign in twenty-five years, took part in dramatic events in Quebec, and organized an exchange visit with Russia, then a shadowy, somewhat forbidden Communist superpower. In addition, Stanley had to deal with the unexpected early retirement of Purse in 1980 and finally, the singular special event for which the CNIB is perhaps best known — a court-ordered benefit concert by the Rolling Stones.

Stanley, like his predecessors, rose to the challenges. By 1979, the library department was struggling to respond to an ever-increasing demand for audio services. Almost two hundred volunteers, working an average of three hours per week, were producing educational texts, job-support materials, and Canadian books and magazines not readily available to visually impaired people from other sources. Still, they could not keep up with demand, and the days of the old Clarke and Smith playback machines were numbered as they had become outdated technology.

Ed Brown, the head librarian, was transferred to the national office to develop the new technical aids program. (During George Beck's presidency, a major study of the library operation had been undertaken and improvements recommended in the Bowron report. It fell to Stanley and Purse to consider how that study, and the Greenland report, should be implemented.)

The energetic and dynamic Françoise Hébert, director of CNIB library services, was hired as a change agent. A progressive, dynamic thinker and exceptionally capable, she brought an outspoken style and outgoing manner that came as a shock to the staid CNIB leadership, but she forged ahead with her agenda.

The CNIB had not held a capital campaign since 1953 when money was raised to build the BakerWood campus. Purse now invited Bill Daniels, CEO of Shell Canada, to chair a campaign. Malcolm (Mac) Stewart and Carl Webber of Toronto volunteered to assist CNIB management, and within a year, $2.6 million had been collected and the conversion of the library's collection to a new, improved cassette system for audio books was well underway.

The question arose of what to do with the thousands of Clarke

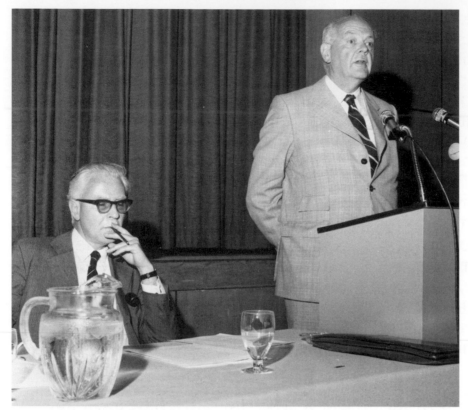

Former president George Beck speaks at the annual general meeting, 1977, while the current president, David Stanley, looks on.

and Smith machines and tens of thousands of tapettes that had brought so much pleasure and information to blind people in Canada. Serviceable machines were refurbished, and they, along with the tapettes, were carefully packaged and shipped to the Caribbean, where it was hoped they would be put to good use.

The CNIB had maintained an ongoing relationship with the Caribbean Council for the Blind (CCB) since the post-war years. Baker had travelled through the region by steamship while conducting a survey of blind people, and blind people from Caribbean countries had attended training programs in Toronto, thanks to financial assistance provided by the federal government.

So while providing an instant audio library to blind people in the Caribbean seemed like a good idea, unfortunately the machines were left to rust in a dockside warehouse and eventually had to be destroyed. The well-meaning Canadians hadn't realized that electrical power was in short supply and of a different standard, no effective distribution system had been set up, and the CCB's resources were limited. Lesson learned.

The four-track cassette system introduced in the 1970s gave reliable service to blind readers for twenty-five years until it, in its turn, was replaced by the next generation of technology, the digital audio book. By the 1990s, books could be stored on compact discs and played on sophisticated, streamlined playback machines that were much easier to use, and another campaign was launched to once again convert the library's collection to another format — from cassette to CD, the fourth generation of the audio book in sixty years.

The success of the capital campaign created two lasting changes in the institute's corporate culture. First, it brought everyone together in a collective national exercise and restored confidence in the institute's image and ability to be a major player on the national stage.

The second change was more significant. Government and United Appeal funding was not enough to keep up with the growing demand for service. CaterPlan was no longer the cash cow it had been, due to increasing competition. From here on, the CNIB would have to be in permanent fundraising mode.

THE ROLLING STONES CONCERT

About this time, a golden publicity opportunity presented itself in the unlikely guise of Keith Richards, lead guitarist with the Rolling Stones. Arriving in Toronto in February 1977 to perform a few club dates at the El Mocambo, the thirty-four-year-old Richards was arrested when an RCMP search of his hotel room turned up one ounce of heroin with a street value of $4,000.

Facing an extremely serious charge of trafficking in heroin, which carried with it a penalty of seven years to life imprisonment, Richards and his Rolling Stones team took the situation very seriously. The case dragged on for a year, and in the end, Richards narrowly escaped jail, partly due to the pleas of a young blind woman who told the court how Richards had made sure she was returned home safely after a Stones concert. He worked out a plea bargain that included a benefit show for the Canadian National Institute for the Blind, which was held April 22, 1979, at the Oshawa Civic Auditorium. Although the sentencing applied only to Richards, the rest of the band, including Mick Jagger, supported their bandmate by performing with him at two sold-out shows.

More than thirteen hundred visually impaired people were given free passes for themselves and a sighted guide, and the rest of the tickets (seventy-four hundred) were sold to the public. The concert raised $50,000 for the CNIB. In accepting the cheque, Bill Milton, assistant managing director of professional development and client services, said the money would be used by CNIB "to help young blind people." Ultimately, the money was allocated to Toronto's Hospital for Sick Children for research into juvenile diabetes, a leading cause of blindness in people under forty.

(Saying he "never had a problem with drugs, only with cops," Richards then decamped for the United States where he underwent drug treatment.)

However, what could have been a potentially lucrative opportunity with spectacular media implications took on a very different life. Vocal blind people viewed the event as gratuitous and condescending, and as for the CNIB leadership, council members expressed concerns ranging from liability issues to the damage that could be done to the CNIB's image by its association with a pot-smoking rock star. The internal dissension became the media event, and William Petryniak, who had been newly hired to bolster financial operations, was left to handle the media. Although well qualified for the job he was hired to do, he had no media relations training or experience, as became evident when he was featured on a national TV news program.

PURSE AND THE AGM

Purse, however, had weightier matters on his mind than a British rock band. The Quebec government had decided to implement its own service programs for its ten thousand blind citizens. Purse went to Quebec City to try to negotiate, but the government remained firm, and he took the difficult decision to close all but three offices that were strategically situated around the province. Less than fifteen years later, only a small office, with about a dozen staff, would remain in Montreal.

The CNIB annual general meeting, always a large, well-attended event, was held in late spring, usually May, at BakerWood. Volunteers and management from across Canada attended, and they were often joined by international guests.

In 1976, Sir John Wilson, a principal founder of the Royal Commonwealth Society for the Blind, was a featured speaker. Wilson had met Colonel Baker at a conference in London, and on an afternoon cruise on the Thames, the two men drew up the constitution of the Royal Commonwealth Society, which assisted blind people in Africa, India, and other countries with ties to Britain. As a result of his work in blindness prevention in developing countries, the World Health Organization dedicated World Health Day 1977 to blindness prevention. Sir John won the support of forty-four countries that agreed to set up a program during the year. The CNIB and the Canadian Ophthalmological Society called a meeting of many organizations — health, government, and community services — and set up the Canadian Coordinating Committee for Blindness Prevention

(CCCOBP). Purse was elected its first chairman. (The Royal Commonwealth Society for the Blind is now known as Sight Savers International. The CCCOBP was short-lived, and it would be many years before another similar group would come together.)

It was around the time of the 1976 AGM that the last surviving founder of the CNIB died. Dr.

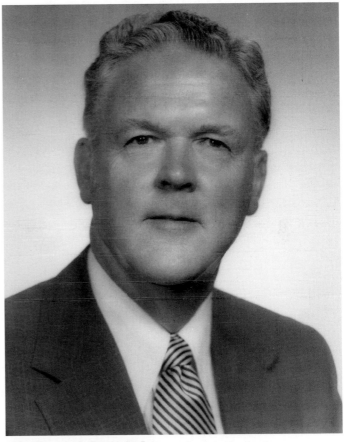

Richard Smith.

261

Charles Watty Carruthers, a lawyer and osteopath, passed away on May 14, 1976.

At the 1979 AGM Richard (Dick) Smith was elected president, only the third person from outside Toronto to hold that position. President of the Smith Agency Limited, a real estate and insurance firm, Smith began as a CNIB volunteer in Manitoba in 1962. He served as chair of the Manitoba division board from 1974 to 1979, when he was elected to National Council.

Colonel Boris Zimin, president of the World Council for the Welfare of the Blind and of the Central Board of the All-Russia Association of the Blind, along with three Soviet colleagues, attended the CNIB's sixty-first AGM in 1979. During his speech, Zimin stressed the need for worldwide understanding and acceptance of visually impaired people. His two-week visit to Canada also included an in-depth tour of the BakerWood complex and visits to CNIB offices in Hamilton, Ottawa, and Montreal. This was the culmination of an exchange begun in October 1978 when Purse and other senior staff members had travelled to the USSR.

It was in Moscow that Purse had told council chair David Stanley, for reasons of his own that were never made public, that he would like to take early retirement. Stanley agreed to negotiate the terms, and in September 1980, Purse stepped down from the CNIB presidency after serving for seven years.

His CNIB career had spanned thirty-three years. Purse relocated to the lower mainland of British Columbia, where he and his wife, Vivian, enjoyed successful careers as real estate agents before again retiring. Despite experiencing prolonged trauma as a prisoner of war, which led to residual health problems, Purse was sustained by his strength of character, self–discipline, and the tremendous support of his wife.

Purse received several personal honors to mark his career and contributions, including the Ambrose M. Shotwell Distinguished Service Award, which was presented to him at the conference of the American Association of Workers for the Blind in 1979. In 1980, the CNIB's National Council established the Ross C. Purse Doctoral Fellowship in recognition of his enduring interest in education. The annual fellowship is awarded for post-graduate special studies and research into the non-medical impact and aspects of blindness.

The process to recruit Purse's successor, the fifth managing director, was a departure from previous practice. CNIB President David Stanley, his successor Richard Smith of Winnipeg, and Dudley Mendels of Montreal were appointed as the search committee; internal and external candidates were interviewed. The process was certainly confidential, if not in fact secretive.

The choice of Robert Mercer, the committee's recommended candidate, was approved by council and he assumed the duties of the CNIB's managing director on September 1, 1980.

ROBERT MERCER

A Nova Scotian from Cape Breton, Robert Mercer attended the Halifax School for the Blind and later St. Mary's University. He had been active in the blind rights and consumer movements as a founder and leader of the Blind Rights Action Movement in Nova Scotia.

When Purse met Mercer in Halifax, he determined that Mercer was a natural leader with a quick, bright mind and challenged him to join the CNIB and improve the organization from within. Mercer agreed, and in 1975 he was appointed as assistant director of the Maritime division; later the

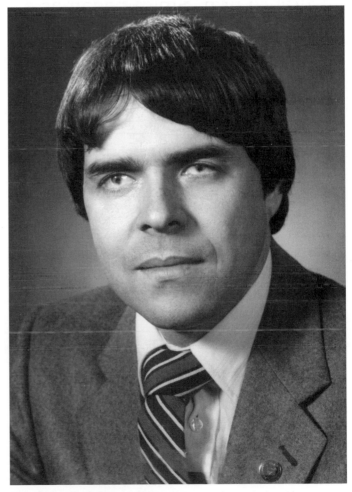

Robert Mercer.

same year he was named executive director of the Saskatchewan division. Two years later he was transferred to the B.C.-Yukon division as executive director, where he remained until his appointment to the national office in Toronto in September 1979 as executive assistant to the managing director.

The CNIB's trustees judged Mercer's youth, energy, and innate business acumen to be right for the times. Also at this time, the decision was made to transfer Euclid Herie, who had been with the CNIB only three years as the executive director in Manitoba, from Winnipeg to Toronto to take up a new position as assistant managing director, replacing William Milton, who was appointed national consultant to senior management. Neither Herie nor Mercer had any say in the matter, but fortunately for both men, the arrangement worked well.

One of Herie's first assignments after arriving in Toronto in January 1980 was to restructure the programs at the A.V. Weir Centre. The residential component was closed, personnel training programs were streamlined, and rehabilitation staff were trans-ferred to the Ontario division to replace the cumbersome purchase of service arrangement from the national office. Within a year of Herie's arrival in Toronto, Mercer asked him to lead the Ontario division on an interim basis. Meanwhile, developments in the Quebec division were unfolding quickly, due mostly to three escalating, volatile labour disputes, a ballooning operating deficit, and a tempestuous board impatient for action. Herie, who was fully bilingual, directed both divisions for two years.

Mercer recruited Gary Magarrell to fill the vacant executive director position in British Columbia. Magarrell became the second sighted external director at Mercer's senior management table. If a new look to the organization in this era was required, Mercer was ready to oblige.

In January 1980, National Council had commissioned a report "to evaluate the efficiency of the present organizational structure of the CNIB," and Mercer was assigned to write it. By the time the report was submitted to council in November 1980, Mercer had become the managing director.

The Mercer report, as it became known, featured several interesting recommendations. It suggested that all national office staff be located in the A.V. Weir Centre, and that the national office be renamed the National Centre for Research and Consultation on Blindness. It recommended that the CNIB library should be given the status of a separate division of the CNIB and no longer be considered merely a department of the national office. It also suggested that direct services to blind people be transferred from the A.V. Weir Centre to the Ontario Division, that the A.V. Weir Centre residence and cafeteria facilities be closed, and that a national department of rehabilitation be created to incorporate the staff and function of the following separate national departments: adjustment to blindness, social services and rehabilitation, employment services, prevention of blindness and eye service, children and youth, war blinded and blind veterans' services. It concluded with the ideas that the Ontario Division and national office negotiate a new relationship, and that a new funding formula be created for the national office.

Mercer believed that locating the national office in the A.V. Weir Centre, away from the Ontario division and the library, would position it as a separate entity. The renovations cost in the order of $600,000, which depleted the national office's Division Assistance Plan.

He had decided that the library operation, with a budget of $1,784,500 in 1980 serving eleven thousand clients, had outgrown the national office management capabilities, and he recommended that the library be re-established as a division, with its own board of management and responsibility for its own financial and operating priorities. Amid considerable debate and controversy, the decision was adopted in November 1980. A less public rationale for creating the ninth division was that as a separate national entity, the library would have more latitude to raise funds from the public for its high-profile service.

Existing agreements with some 130 United Appeals placed serious restrictions on supplementary fundraising activities in urban communities. The library, it was argued, would have no such limitations. And although it was rumoured that eventually the library would become financially autonomous and independent, this was never in the Mercer plan.

What soon became evident was the resistance of the eight geographic sibling divisions to the arrival of the CNIB's new baby. Up to now, divisions had funded library services on a per capita assessment based on the number of subscribers. That, too, was problematic because the more library users registered with a division, the higher its library assessment. Obviously, this meant divisions dragged their feet in promoting library services to new clients and were not quick to sign up new subscribers.

In the crunch of annual budgeting and scarce dollars, this sizable line item was a tempting target. Although stoutly denied, the practice went on for many years until the funding formula was changed to a universal assessment based on the total clients registered.

But the problems did not end there. The library division had been created equal to the others — able to set annual operating priorities and budget. Once these had been approved, funding came from the assessments and contracts for production with little fundraising to offset costs. Inevitably, the library incurred sizable operating deficits that had to be funded by subsidies from national reserve funds. The national office, which was funded by the provincial divisions for both capital and operating needs, levied assessments on the divisions, which, in the end, funded any unfunded portion of the library budget. The depletion of the national office's Division Assistance Program for the renovation of the A.V. Weir Centre added to the financial malaise. Teetering on the horns of this dilemma, a happy solution remains elusive.

The library operated at a deficit from the beginning, and no capital fund was set up for the library to fulfill capital purchases of computers and costly recording and embossing equipment. This arrangement was not workable and proved divisive to a house that was in many ways already divided.

Gerald Tremblay, a Montreal lawyer who served on the national board, described what was happening succinctly when he said in a 2003 interview, "You have the intolerable situation of one division having the power to tax its sister divisions through the budget process." Tremblay suggested that having one entity, the national office, levying assessments was enough. Moreover, by acting on its new mandate and expectation to pursue creative new fundraising opportunities, the library was treading on the toes of the provinces until they hurt.

Unfazed by these growing pains, Mercer moved forward with his agenda. He released the unfortunate William Petryniak, who had got caught up in the Rolling Stones circus and who had never really been able to get beyond the established power base in Toronto, retired several long-term employees, and gave unprecedented authority and freedom to divisional directors to manage their operations.

Mercer, while not being disrespectful to his predecessors, also brought a more informal style to the cafeteria and boardroom that was in tune with the times. He flattened a hierarchical management structure to make the organization more democratic and to draw in more blind people. He supported Magarrell's push, amid huge controversy, for open board meetings in British Columbia. Well

liked and respected, the affable Mercer was imaginative and fearless. At the time of his appointment, he was not yet thirty.

An example of his innovative thinking was his proposal that the Lake Joseph Holiday Centre be converted into a facility for training guide dogs. This was the only opportunity the CNIB would have to establish such a program. Those who opposed him argued that the Americans had provided the service for fifty years at no charge and thus it was a "met need." Within three years, no fewer than three schools opened in Canada, demonstrating that indeed there was a need. So for the CNIB, that parade had passed. A timid attempt to purchase Canadian Guide Dogs for the Blind, a school located in Manotick, near Ottawa, in the late 1990s was never realized.

Early in his term, Mercer had thought aloud that a national low vision program, comparable to the Lighthouse program in New York, might be established at the A.V. Weir Centre. He failed to anticipate the professional jealousies this idea would spark among the eye health care community. Optometrists, non-medical practitioners with post-graduate specialization in assessing visual function, liked the idea. The Canadian Ophthalmological Society — representing medical doctors who specialize in the diagnosis and treatment of eye disease and who prescribe and administer medication and perform surgery — opposed the concept loudly and vigorously. The debate raged in the media, and Mercer appeared on a national news program to explain the controversy. Knowing full well what he was doing, Mercer had ignited the flash point between the two eye health specialties in Canada that until then had kept their differences, bitter at times, to a local level. Mercer had elevated the discussion to a national forum. In the end, however, the centre was never created.

In April 1983, after serving as CNIB president for three years, Mercer resigned, taking the organization by surprise. In a 2004 interview in Halifax, he discussed his reasons for leaving.

Expressing some frustration, he noted:

> At the time I decided to leave we were at the point where some of the

things that needed to be put in place weren't getting done, like the low vision centre, so that was a disappointment. I don't think the board wanted to be active in pushing things publicly and sometimes you need to do that.

But with hindsight today, I know that the real reason I left was because I had outgrown the job. I never went to the CNIB with the idea that I would be there until I retired; I thought when I joined that I had some knowledge and experience that would be helpful to the organization. But after thirteen years, I was not being challenged and I wasn't learning anymore. Also I was having some medical issues, which were job related, and I was ready to leave.

Mercer went on to a successful career as a civil servant, holding senior positions with the Treasury

Board, Canadian Centre for Management Development, and Veterans Affairs. By CNIB standards, three years was not a long time to be president. But for blind Canadians those three years would prove to be pivotal, changing as they did the course of history in the disability field.

Mercer deserves credit for what he did. As the old farm adage has it, whoever shall take blame for the rain is entitled to take credit for the sunshine — and shine it did.

In 1981, a phone call from Walter Gretzky launched a friendship that would prove to be of great value to the CNIB, both financially and for public awareness and good will. Wayne Gretzky sports tournaments were held annually for eleven summers, and later, Walter's golf tournaments, the establishment of the Walter and Wayne Gretzky Youth Scholarship Fund, and Walter's active support of the SCORE teen computer camps left an enduring legacy.

But perhaps nothing did more to change the world view of disabled people than the United Nations' resolution, which was seconded by Walter Dinsdale of Manitoba, to declare 1981 as International Year of Disabled Persons (IYDP).

The Honourable Monique Bégin, minister of National Health and Welfare, appointed Euclid Herie to Canada's national coordinating committee.

Canadian successes from IYDP included the funding of a national meeting at the CNIB Lake Joseph Centre of deaf-blind people who had no voice of their own. Delegates to the meeting founded the Canadian National Association of Deafblind Persons, which in time joined an international group. Services for deaf-blind Canadians continue to be fragmented.

THE IYDP AND ITS SERIES OF OBSTACLES REPORTS

Because of the heightened awareness of the IYDP, the government of Canada appointed a parliamentary committee on disability to give disabled Canadians a place on the national agenda. Although progress in achieving equality with non-disabled Canadians is still a work in progress, there's no doubt that had it not been for the IYDP, victories, however small, would have taken much longer to achieve.

The next year, 1982, brought what many would regard as a triumph, not only for clients of the CNIB but for all Canadians with disabilities.

Prime Minister Pierre Elliott Trudeau was determined to complete the patriation of the Canadian Constitution, a process that had effectively begun with the signing of the British North America Act in 1867.

As Canada grew in both population and territory, many new challenges faced the federal government. The need for full control of Canadian foreign policy and of the constitutional amending procedure became evident. Steps taken to achieve full patriation included the Statute of Westminster in 1931, the Bill of Rights of 1960, and finally the Constitution of 1982, with its accompanying Charter of Rights and Freedoms.

Conspicuously absent from the draft of the Charter of Rights was any reference to disabilities.

Mercer seized the moment. While success is said to have many parents, the CNIB took a leadership role in this historic process. David Lepofsky, then a twenty-three-year-old blind law student and member of the Ontario Board of Directors, volunteered to act as the CNIB spokesman on matters relating to the Charter of Rights and to draft a submission which the CNIB hoped to present to the government.

On the morning of Friday, February 12, 1980, a small CNIB delegation consisting of Lepofsky, CNIB Managing Director Robert Mercer, and national vice-president Dr. Dayton Forman appeared before the Special Joint Committee on the Constitution of Canada, made up of various government officials and members of the House of Commons and Senate. Besides the CNIB delegation, representatives from the World Federalists of Canada and Operation Dismantle were also present.

After the meeting had been called to order, Dr. Forman introduced Mercer, who briefly described the work of the CNIB and then called on Lepofsky to present the position of the CNIB on the subject of human rights.

But before he got to the main part of his presentation, Lepofsky made a powerful statement on the meaning of equality by asking that braille and audio cassette versions of his brief, which the CNIB delegation had brought with them, be distributed to anyone at the table who might want or require one.

During his presentation Lepofsky described the "well-intentioned cruelty which many members of the public unintentionally or unknowingly impose upon [blind people]." He went on, "The pity, the patronization, discriminatory attitudes and condescension which handicapped people know to be, unfortunately, almost nonstop components of their life, is, in fact, the biggest problem they face."

Lepofsky went on to give examples of discrimination faced by disabled people in the areas of jobs, housing, and access to higher education. He explained that the CNIB was concerned not just with discriminatory human conduct but with "legislation which discriminates." In scholarly legal terms, he made a persuasive argument, citing example after example why "handicapped people are entitled to equality before the law and to the equal protection of the law."

When Lepofsky finished his presentation, several committee members followed up with questions and comments.

In one poignant and telling exchange, Senator John Connolly of Ontario said:

> But I would like to ask Mr. Lepofsky this. You have been talking … about the importance of integrating the handicapped community into the normal stream of public life … I do not ask this as a trick question, but I wonder whether, by segregating the handicapped (that is giving them specific mention in the charter) you are not, to use your own words, signaling to the disabled that they are forever a segregated group?

The CNIB's recommendations were accepted.

Section 15 of Canada's Charter of Rights and Freedom, which leads off the Equality section, reads: "Every individual is equal before and under the law and has the right to the equal protection and equal benefit of the law without discrimination and, in particular, without discrimination based on race, national or ethnic origin, colour, religion, sex, age or mental or physical disability."

Brilliant? Many consider it the CNIB's finest hour.

As for young Lepofsky, the year after his appearance before the Constitution Committee, he earned a master's degree in law from Harvard and went on to a distinguished career with the Ontario government's Ministry of the Attorney General. He remains a passionate advocate for equality and played a key role in the campaign for an Ontarians with Disabilities Act.

CHAPTER 13
The Power of the Dream
by Elizabeth Duncan

In 1983, Euclid Herie was appointed managing director of the CNIB, and over the next seventeen years, as his life's journey took him to some of the most exotic and remote places within Canada and around the world, his message remained the same: it's respectable to be blind.

And it was during the Herie years, building on the experience, reputation, and social conscience of the previous decades, that the Canadian experience of what it means to be blind truly began to change. But like an ocean liner changing direction, the shift came slowly and was the result of driving forces both from within the CNIB and from the external environment.

The son of a farmer father and teacher mother, Herie was born in the poor farming community of St. Jean de Baptiste, Manitoba, in 1939 with congenital cataracts. His vision problems went unnoticed until he was about three, but in those days, in that place, there was no medical treatment available. When he was about sixteen,

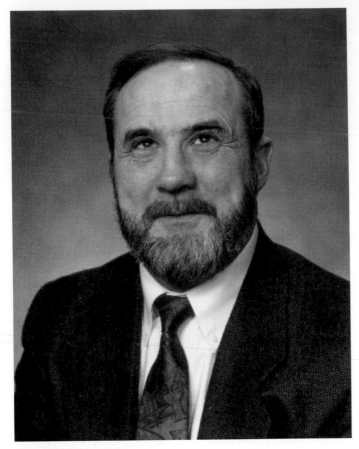

Euclid Herie.

his eyesight failed dramatically in about three days over Christmas, and in February 1956 he was sent into Regina to meet with Ross Purse, who would later become the CNIB's fourth president. Purse arranged for Herie to be registered for a correspondence program so he could finish Grade 10 and then to be sent to the School for the Blind in Brantford for grades 11 and 12. Herie then returned to his home province to continue his education at the University of Manitoba.

His first work experience with the CNIB, stacking sticky pop bottles in a canteen during the summer of 1956, didn't fill him with hope for a long-term future. "I was always motivated to get a good education. I think out of 150 cousins, only two of us got degrees. It just wasn't the culture of the time, in our family."

Herie finished a B.A., and although he would have liked to go into law, he was encouraged to enter the Bachelor of Social Work program, social work being one of the few professions considered suitable for blind people at that time. He landed a job with the Children's Aid Society in Winnipeg in May 1963. In 1965 he earned a master's degree in social work, and he worked for the agency until he was recruited by the CNIB in 1977 as the executive director of the Manitoba division. At a high personal cost to his family, which included two school-age children, and with great reluctance, Herie agreed to move to Toronto in the late fall of 1979 to take up the recently created position of assistant to the new managing director, Robert Mercer. He began this work in January 1980.

For three years, Herie and Mercer worked closely together, handling a variety of problems, including a sexual assault incident at the Lake Joseph Holiday Centre, the accelerated closure of the residences across Canada, and trouble brewing within the Ontario and Quebec divisions as unrest and dissatisfaction increased.

In the summer of 1981, at Mercer's request, Herie took over running the Ontario division, and in the early winter of 1982, after the problems in Quebec described earlier began to escalate, he also took over the running of the Quebec division, all the while maintaining his national office workload. "I went back and forth from Toronto to Montreal about thirty-five times in six months. I was on the road for an entire year. It was extremely difficult. I was never home. I once figured out that in twenty-five years at the CNIB I lived in hotels for eleven years."

By February 1983, exhausted and approaching burnout, Herie decided to take a vacation, so he persuaded his wife, Ellen, who didn't like flying, to go to Mexico.

The night we got back, while we're still unpacking the souvenirs, I got a call from Robert Mercer, who said he needed to speak to me, and would I meet him in the coffee shop of the Prince Hotel. I wasn't happy about this. It was a Sunday night, I had just got back from a short vacation, and I thought here we go again, we're already back into it.

I had pretty well decided that for lots of reasons, not least of which I was killing myself, that I was going to leave the CNIB. I'd had enough. [Because of the situation in Quebec] I was living under police protection, my family had been threatened, I had to register in hotels under false names and I had faced a lot of grief with the Ontario boards. It was all very unpleasant.

So I told my wife, "I'm going to meet with Bob and when I get back, I'll have told him I'm leaving the CNIB."

Bob and I talked about Mexico for a few minutes, and then he said he was calling a meeting for the next morning to announce his resignation. I said, "That's odd because I came to tell you I'm leaving."

I certainly wasn't thinking, "Oh good, now I can have the top job," I was thinking I would be leaving, too.

But apparently, a select group of council members held a meeting at the Granite Club on Bayview Avenue and I got a call from Jack Pequegnat, chairman of the Ontario Board of Management, asking if he could come over and talk to me about the managing director's position, and he said if we could come to an understanding, the appointment would be effective May 1, 1983.

When I joined the CNIB in 1977 and came to Toronto in 1979 it was never in my wildest imagination that I would be the CNIB managing director, or president as the job title later became.

A relentlessly inquisitive man who examines everything that crosses his path in great detail, Herie is sensitive to the environment around him and doesn't miss much.

On reflection, he feels that the expectations for his predecessor, Robert Mercer, had been too high.

He had a lot to deal with, he was dynamic, he would be the new man, the new image, he presented well, he was articulate, and he was leading the CNIB into a new era and that's what they wanted. But I think what happened, in part, is when they got it, it was more than they anticipated and maybe it happened too fast, but Robert was that kind of guy. He was doing exactly what he was expected to do, but maybe he did in two years what should have taken five.

When he did leave, there was bad blood and I had to face that with the trustees.

In 1983, Dr. Gerald E. Dirks, a blind professor of political science at Brock University, was hired to be the interim executive director of the Ontario division, taking those direct responsibilities off Herie's shoulders.

At the time of Herie's appointment as managing director, 40,858 blind and visually impaired people were registered with the CNIB, and the operating budget was almost $49 million. A strategic thinker and planner with astute political instincts, Herie rolled up his sleeves and went to work. And as events unfolded, the impetus for all the changes that occurred during his tenure would seem to have been a natural consequence of the empowerment movements of the 1960s and '70s.

CLOSING THE RESIDENCES AND WORKSHOPS

One of the biggest issues facing the CNIB in the 1980s was the sale of some of its buildings and the closure of the residences and workshops, all of which were located in prime real estate locations and were deeply entrenched in their communities. None of them went quietly, and there was always disagreement and dissension as feelings ran high. Among the properties sold were Quinte St. Lawrence Hall in Kingston, Tweedsmuir Hall in London, Huronia Hall in Kitchener, and Linwell Hall in St. Catharines.

In the B.C.-Yukon division, the sale of property was conducted amid massive negative publicity. Through a shrewd negotiation led by Captain M.C. Robinson, national director, Western Canada, the CNIB had obtained Queen Elizabeth Hall and its surrounding parkland in a deal with the City of

Vancouver. In the mid-1990s the CNIB sold the property to a developer for more than $6 million; the profit on the sale led to the CNIB's being labelled "greedy" in media headlines.

By 1990, fifteen additional residences had been phased out, leaving only three, in Hamilton, St. John's, and Cornerbrook. The summer camps at Bowen Island in British Columbia and Lake Joseph in Ontario managed to elude Herie; he would have liked to have sold them off, but they remain CNIB property. Nowhere did a building's closure attract more negative media attention or cause feelings to run higher than when ClarkeWood, the CNIB's flagship residence on Bayview Avenue in Toronto, was torn down in 1993, which happened to be the organization's seventy-fifth anniversary year. The building had been closed several years earlier.

The perception in the media, recalled Herie, was of:

> … the mean CNIB putting all these poor blind people out on the street and cutting off their livelihoods … But the truth for the residences was that blind people had long since stopped coming to them. In fact, some of the residences, like Sudbury and Quebec City, had empty beds from the day they opened and in many cases we were taking sighted people to get the bed count full because the funding had changed. Still, it was a very emotional time.

The residences had grown old along with the people they housed. Most of the buildings no longer conformed to codes, and the residents, many of whom had come to the residence in their forties, were now in their eighties, and their needs had changed.

Some of the residences had workshops attached, so they were phased out, too. By 1990, many workshops were gone, leaving only a small program in Calgary and three programs in Ontario (in Sudbury, Hamilton, and Toronto). These closures marked the end of an era in employment that had spanned well over a century. The last workshop to close was the broom shop, located on the lower level of the CNIB building in Toronto, which ceased operations in 2001.

The situation in Quebec was different. Working with John Avon, a highly respected pioneer in employment and training for the blind, Herie was able to negotiate the sale of workshop operations in Montreal and Quebec City to a consortium of blind workers. A similar attempt to save the broom shop in Toronto failed. The downside to closing the residences and selling off buildings was the loss of a CNIB presence in the communities it served. Herie recalled:

> Long before I joined the CNIB there was that big building on the corner of Portage and Sherburn [in Winnipeg] — it was a landmark since the 1920s. There was this great white cane — I often wondered where that went, by the way — all lit up at night with the red CNIB neon sign, about a story high. You had the Blindcraft store where they sold women's dresses, you could go by the residence next door, which was a nice, scenic walk and you had all these contented old blind people sitting in their chairs after dinner.
>
> Also there was what I think was the first audible crossing signal, which had been installed by the 1950s, so blind people could cross the road safely. That bell and buzzer system was known to every driver in Winnipeg who drove along Portage Avenue.
>
> So if you take the high profile that building had, apply that recognition to dozens of other communities across Canada which had major buildings, this was the community awareness level the CNIB enjoyed. By the way, I think this local presence led to a lot of bequests for the CNIB because the perception was we were taking good care of blind people.

As the residences were closed, the CNIB replaced them with new service centres, which provided a different level and kind of care. The CNIB began to promote independence and the concept of blind people thriving in a sighted world. Herie opened at least twenty new service centres across Canada.

THE TECHNOLOGY REVOLUTION

As early as 1974, when a blind physicist at the University of Oxford in England developed an electronic calculator with audio output, technology began to change the world for blind people, and the CNIB was quick to realize the potential both for itself and its clients.

By 1976 the CNIB had acquired a Honeywell computer and brought in a Data General machine. Managing Director Robert Mercer, amid great controversy, persuaded the board to purchase a mainframe computer that filled a huge room, with the intention that it would be used to computerize some of the accounting functions and the client database. Although the mainframe operation was eventually shut down, a report commissioned at the time determined that the CNIB had "spent its money wisely" in respect to its early adoption of computerization. The first installation in the world of the Duxbury Translator, a software program used to print braille, took place at the CNIB in July 1976. In 1974, Gulf Canada presented the CNIB with one of the first reading machines invented by Raymond Kurzweil of Kurzweil Applied Intelligence in Massachusetts.

Herie recalled:

> They used to move it on a dolly over to the auditorium. The thing looked like two steamer trunks and it did read, sort of, it could read certain fonts, but it was the first reading machine. So we saw the first years of what we now call adaptive technology and we were far from the day of the readable scanners, laptops, refreshable braille, and accessible technology that was coming, but CNIB was definitely in on that from the beginning.

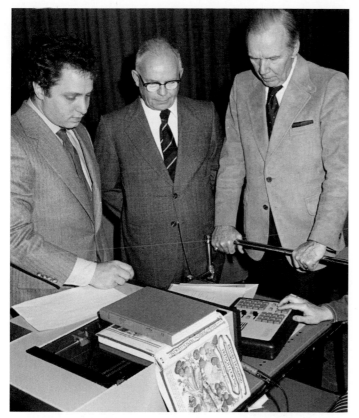

Managing Director Ross Purse (right) and Mr. Harris, president of Gulf Canada, inspect the Kurzweil Reader, 1974. The person on the left is unknown.

ming in this country, and a lot of them were very successful with the federal government and private industry. And what's more, a few of them were women.

When Herie became managing director, he made technology a priority. A small technology unit was set up in the A.V. Weir Centre, one was planned for Winnipeg, and the divisions were asking for hands-on, walk-in technology catalogues.

By 1985 computers had been introduced into all nine operating divisions for financial and human service data, and the library's circulation system had been automated. Micro-computers, as they were called, were being used to transform print into braille. Also in 1985, the CNIB Technology Task Force, composed of senior staff, management, and board members, submitted a proposed policy to National Council. Its acceptance created the new Technical Aids Service, which would play a major role in the years to come. CNIB staff took on the additional role of training clients to use screen reading and voice output technology,

And you have to remember that around this time there were a lot of blind computer programmers, who were probably in the vanguard of computer program-which could transform their ability to access the printed word.

By the 1990s, with the introduction of specialized software programs, blind or sighted volunteers could use the new technology to translate French or music braille. To encourage innovation in technological advances that would benefit blind people, in 1988 the CNIB, under the leadership of National Council President Tim Sheeres, inaugurated the Winston Gordon Award for Technological Advancement in the Field of Blindness and Visual Impairment. Named in memory of a long-time friend and benefactor to the CNIB, the award includes a gold medal and a generous cash prize. Sheeres continued to maintain a keen interest in the Winston Gordon Award program, and as of 2004 remains chair of its selection committee.

On March 30, 1993, after three years of planning under the direction of Robert Elton, director of communications and human resources, and funded in part by a $200,000 grant from Transport Canada, the CNIB launched the Technibus to celebrate its seventy-fifth anniversary. With coordinators Lydia Bardak and Carrie Anton on board, the twelve-metre bus travelled thirty-eight thousand kilometres across Canada, through all ten provinces and one territory, bringing examples of the latest in high and low technology to blind and visually impaired people who otherwise might not have access to a CNIB centre. It was believed to be the world's first mobile technology exhibit. Many of the seventeen thousand visitors to the bus said it was the first time they had had the opportunity to experience and examine technical aids that could make a difference in their lives ... everything from self-threading needles and large print playing cards to optical scanners that could read text.

As for Kurzweil's reading machine, by 1993, the year of the Technibus Odyssey, it worked 80 times faster, contained 128 times the memory, was 1/26th the price of the original model, and had a fancier name, The Reading Edge.

Fran Cutler, CNIB chair from 2000 to 2003, says it's impossible to underestimate the impact of computer technology on the lives of people who are blind or

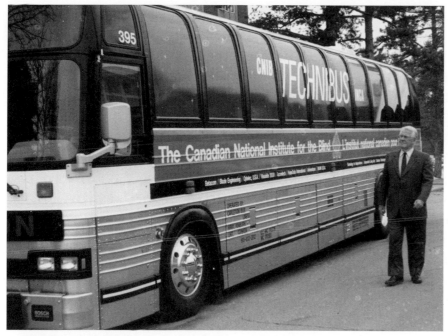

CNIB President Robert Waugh inspects the Technibus.

SEE POLICY

In 1985 the CNIB undertook a major change in the services it provided. Since its founding in 1918, it had worked to ameliorate the condition of blind people across Canada and to prevent blindness. In 1985 a third objective was added to its mandate: "To provide sight enhancement services." Based on a year-long study and consultations undertaken by Charlene Muller, blindness prevention coordinator, National Council authorized a task force to develop a plan of action — and from this, Sight Enhancement Enterprise (SEE) was born. SEE was a program for all people seeking help because of failing or poor vision. Often a person's visual impairment is not enough to be considered blindness, as the term is usually defined, but is serious enough to cause problems with employment, reading, driving, and recognizing faces.

This policy change meant that access to CNIB services would no

visually impaired. "It was really the third step on the access to information path for people who are blind or visually impaired," she says. "First, there was braille in the 1830s, then recorded sound in the first half of the twentieth century, and now the computer era. By extending the range of services to include computer technology, the CNIB has enriched the lives of hundreds of thousands of Canadians."

longer be exclusive to people who were blind. The program, which was set up with a five-year budget of $6.5 million, was designed to help either by assisting the person directly or by facilitating referral to an appropriate community service. CNIB was able to expand services to people with low vision. Staff were trained to assess how clients were using their remaining vision and to provide training in the use of low vision aids such as hand-held magnifiers, telescopes, and, later, computers.

Although the SEE policy was implemented on Herie's watch, he didn't like it.

Why is CNIB in the low vision business? Visually impaired people should be able to go to their eye specialists and low vision clinics that more properly belong in health science centres. If you read the 1984 policy when we established sight enhancement as a priority, as a new found-ing objective, the whole policy stated that, where practical, CNIB low vision services would be incorporated into health science centres, but this never happened.

And also, the CNIB was founded to serve blind people. So when you mix in the low vision population, the question becomes, "How blind are you?"

The Canadian Council of the Blind, a blindness advocacy group, also opposed the SEE policy, say-ing it would diminish the quality of services available to the blind.

FORMATION OF THE NEW BRUNSWICK DIVISION

From 1919 to 1986, CNIB services in New Brunswick, Nova Scotia, and Prince Edward Island had been delivered from Halifax in what was called the Maritime division. In the 1980s, the government of New Brunswick decided it would no longer send money to Halifax to support CNIB services, so Fundy Hall in Saint John, which had been bequeathed to the CNIB, was sold for $200,000. After two years of difficult and sometimes acrimonious negotiating to determine how assets should be divided, the job was finally done, and in January 1986, New Brunswick became the CNIB's tenth operating division, with five district offices offering bilingual services.

CORE SERVICES

In 1985 Herie introduced the concept of strategic planning, which prompted the CNIB to take a closer look at who it was and what it did. What services were being delivered? What services should be delivered? How can we get from here to there?

To help answer some of these questions, in 1988 the service equity task force prioritized CNIB services and designated seven core rehabilitation and library services.

1. Counselling and referral to anyone concerned about poor or failing vision, or who is blind. This includes the parents of blind children, youths and adults. [In the mid-1990s, the CNIB client base would be broken down into three main client groups: children, working age adults, and seniors, all of whom have different needs for different stages of their lives. No matter the person's age or extent of vision loss, dealing with the emotional aspects is a huge challenge.]

2. Orientation and Mobility training for safe and independent travel with the white cane or a guide dog. [The CNIB is not affiliated with a guide dog school nor does it provide training for working with a guide dog. Candidates for guide dogs, however, need to have mastered the orientation and mobility skills taught by CNIB staff.]

3. Rehabilitation teaching to enable persons to acquire independent skills in home management, activities of daily living, leisure and communica-

tions, including braille instruction.

4. Sight enhancement services to assist persons with residual vision to make effective use of the vision they have left, including the use of low vision aids such as magnifying glasses, lighting, glare control through hats and sun glasses, and ensuring high contrast in the living environment, such as black on white signage.

5. Technical Aids programs for daily living, at home, at work, at play.

6. Library services in English braille, French and English talking books and magazines, braille music and job or school support in both braille and recorded format. Also available to clients is the Information Resource Centre, the library without walls, which provides information and research assistance to clients and CNIB staff.

7. Career Development and Employment services assist working age clients to become job ready and advise employers on workplace adaptation and in breaking down attitudinal barriers.

Once prioritized, the question became how to deliver these services uniformly throughout Canada, so every blind person would have equal access to them. After many studies and much debate, from a dozen names resulting from a focus group — and without any consensus — Herie and National Council President Tim Sheeres declared that this new concept would be called "service equity." By 2000 the organization was still struggling with what service equity meant, as it tried to deliver service to more clients with financial resources decreasing.

FROM MANAGING DIRECTOR TO PRESIDENT

In the 1980s, the CNIB's fundraising efforts took on a new dimension when the organization got into gaming, including weekend casino operations, monster bingos, and lotteries. President John R. Baker, son of CNIB co-founder Edwin Baker, opposed this shift in the corporate culture, saying if his father had been alive, he never would have allowed the CNIB to get into gaming. Herie disagreed, saying Baker would have allowed it because it was bringing in badly needed funds.

In 1987, Baker completed a five-year term as CNIB president, and when he left office, in an extraordinarily moving gesture, he presented his father's civil and military medals to the CNIB. Baker died in 1996 in King City, Ontario. Baker was succeeded by Tim Sheeres, who served as president of National Council from 1987 to 1992.

Trained as a chartered accountant in England, Sheeres was recruited in 1975 to serve on the national finance committee, and following early retirement from a successful career in the oil and gas industry, based in Calgary and Toronto, he devoted many hours to the CNIB. In 1990, the CNIB updated its naming conventions. Tim Sheeres, president of the organization's governing body, National Council, became chairman, and Euclid Herie, managing director, became president and chief executive officer. National Council retained that name for a few more years, but by 1997 it had become the CNIB Board of Directors.

Sheeres served until 1992 but continued to maintain an active interest in the organization and for many years attended every important event, videotaping the proceedings for posterity. Sheeres's successor, Robert Waugh, was born in Hamilton, graduated from McMaster University, served in the navy during the Second World War, and had a distinguished career with General Motors Corp. in Canada and the United States. An active volunteer in not-for-profit organizations, he was invited to join the finance committee of CNIB in 1987, became chair of the committee the following year, and went on to become chair of National Council in 1992.

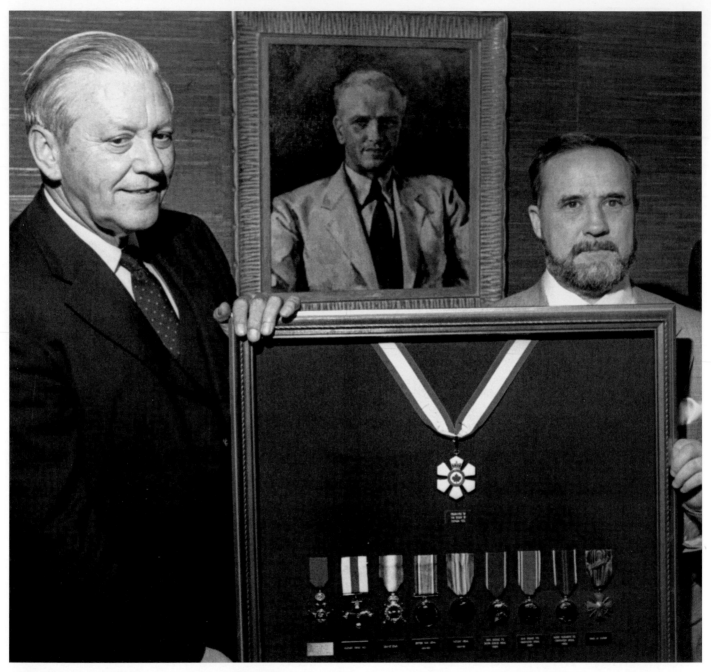

CNIB President John Baker (left) presents his father's medals to Euclid Herie.

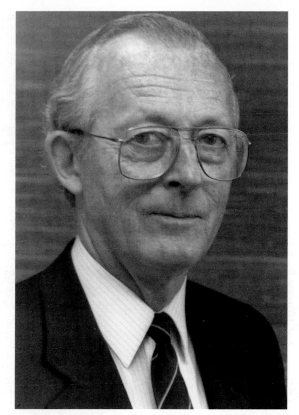

Tim Sheeres.

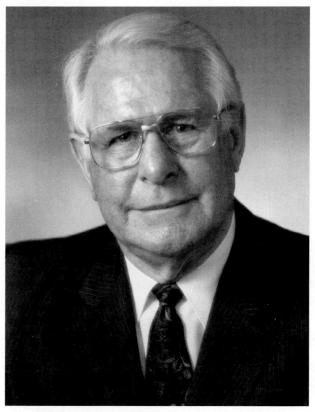

Robert Waugh.

During Waugh's time in office Canada was experiencing a prolonged economic recession that was causing the institute great concern. "The need for sound governance was being increasingly recognized and the divisions had been allowed to develop their own financing and standards for accounting," Waugh said. "These were tough times and we were concerned about our overall finan-cial situation so to make governance more practical, we set out to standardize the financial situation across country, and encourage consistent investment and auditing policies." Part of that was driven by the need to find savings so that led to people working on what became known as the balanced budget and adequate resources policy. A couple of divisions were providing good service and had more funding than they needed, so they allowed the national office to transfer some of these funds to more needy divisions. (This procedure, so casually begun, came into full and formal effect in 2001 as the Hochhausen revenue sharing formula.)

The process, however, while it seemed like a good idea, had serious drawbacks, Waugh believed, and led to much discussion over revenue-sharing formulae that should be used to ensure service equity throughout the country.

"Ontario raised more money, and had proportionately more clients. In my opinion, moving money from the have divisions to have not, merely brought the haves down to the level of the have nots, and relieved the have nots from some of their fundraising responsibilities to the point where the financial strength of the Institute was weakened," Waugh said. Considered as have-not divisions were Atlantic Canada, Saskatchewan, Quebec, and later B.C.-Yukon. After three years, which was as long as he wanted to serve, Waugh stepped down, and in 1995 Calgary lawyer Gary Homer became the CNIB's chairman. He was only the fourth person from outside Ontario to serve in this position.

Born and raised in Newfoundland, Homer practised law in Calgary, where he became involved with the Lions, and through that association in the mid-1960s he met people in the CNIB and was invited to serve on Alberta boards, which led to his being offered a place on the National Council.

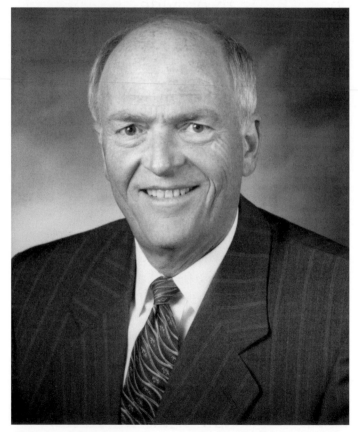

Gary Homer.

As the theme of his five-year tenure as national chairman, Homer chose the analogy of the three-legged stool: the organization was built on a foundation of communication, service, and finances. "We had to recognize that the CNIB, steeped in history and tradition, was also a charity and it had to move with the times," Homer said. "My position was that the role and function of the CNIB is to provide service and how well it can do that depends on how much money it has, and how much money it can raise depends on how well known it is in the community of people who are prepared to financially assist it."

INTERNATIONAL WORK

Although all of Herie's predecessors, from E.A. Baker to Robert Mercer, had attended meetings of international associations of the blind, none of them had a place on the world blindness stage like Herie did.

The World Blind Union (WBU) is the only organization entitled to speak on behalf of blind and partially sighted people of the world, representing 180 million blind and visually impaired people from about 600 different organizations in 158 countries. The WBU was created at a conference in Riyadh, Saudi Arabia, in 1984 when the World Council for the Welfare of the Blind and the International Federation of the Blind voted to form a single world body, the WBU, divided into seven regions. In 1984, the North America/Caribbean region elected William Gallagher, executive director of the American Foundation for the Blind, as its first president. Within a year, Herie's mentor and longtime friend Kenneth Jernigan had succeeded Gallagher and served as the regional president until just before his death in October 1998. Jernigan, a powerful spokesman for the rights of the blind, was for many years a leader at the National Federation of the Blind, based in Baltimore, Maryland.

In 1988, at the second WBU General Assembly held in Madrid, Herie was elected treasurer, a position he held for eight years. He described his involvement:

And like the CNIB, it never occurred to me

that I would be the world president. And then a funny series of events took place.

In the run up to the 1996 General Assembly, which was scheduled to be held in Hong Kong, huge problems began to emerge. Some were political, between the different blindness organizations, and the costs were going to be prohibitive so with less than a year to go, it was decided the assembly could not be held in Hong Kong.

The two countries that bid were New Zealand and Canada, and with a 10–2 vote for Toronto, Canada was chosen.

I had pretty well decided that eight years with the WBU was enough, it was a lot of work and there had been a cost to the CNIB for me to do it.

One day Tim [Sheeres] and I went up to Bob Waugh's cottage and as we were having a sandwich, Bob asked, "How would you like to be the president of the World Blind Union?"

But it wasn't as simple as that. North America only had twelve votes out of about four hundred, so to get elected you needed Africa, Europe, Asia, so we decided to set up a war cabinet and be strategic. [CNIB vice-presidents] Gerrard Grace, Gary Magarrell, and Jim Sanders played a big role in this, and through the network we had we were able to mount a campaign. However, at the last minute the opposition candidate withdrew so I was acclaimed.

I think having the WBU Assembly in Toronto in 1996 changed the course of the CNIB; it brought huge spinoffs. The CNIB put a lot of effort into this and it was done with class. It brought together staff and volunteers — not across the country — but in Toronto and I think it was the best thing the CNIB did in thirty years.

Organizing the logistics of the Fourth General Assembly, attended by 600 delegates and observers from 150 countries over 10 days, placed enormous demands on CNIB staff.

The communications team, guided by board member and former CBC producer Fran Cutler and led by National Director of Communications Marilyn Rewak, generated award-winning media coverage on a scale unlike anything the CNIB had ever seen before.

Darleen Bogart, an international expert on braille and senior volunteer, led a team of braillists that produced a mountain of documents for the assembly.

With dedicated, long-time staff members like Carol Putt and Elaine Spicer, a team of volunteers was taught how to guide blind people, and service staff at local restaurants and hotels were instructed on how to serve meals or assist blind people. Events were staged all across Toronto.

Putt later recalled some of the challenges of bringing together blind people from around the world to the WBU assembly. "Some of these people were coming from the poorest countries in the world, and indoor plumbing, with running water, was something they had never experienced before," she said. "Some of them were also reluctant to spend their per diem meal money — they could only think how much they wanted to save it to take home to their families."

The 1996 assembly featured the first WBU blind women's forum, to focus the world's attention on their vulnerability to abuse, neglect, and marginalization and on the sad fact that in many countries, blind girls are denied the right to an education. As the WBU was paying for participants to attend, it asked that half of each country's delegation be women.

By 1996, Herie had been head of the CNIB for thirteen years and had established good working arrangements with field management. "I was confident that the executive directors I had in place knew what they were doing and I was happy to let them get on with their jobs," he said. "The vice presidents were solid, things were manageable, we weren't in financial crisis, the Quebec downsizing was finished, so I was freer to take on the WBU role than I would have been ten years earlier."

Remembered Gary Homer, "The CNIB Board of Directors took the position that the CNIB should be a leader in promoting services for blind people throughout the world, and we'll support you, but don't forget your day job."

Over the course of his WBU presidency, Herie, usually accompanied by his executive assistant Barbara Marjeram, Homer, and his wife, Joan, visited more than sixty countries, giving speeches, promoting women's rights, braille literacy, and technology, meeting with heads of state, and lobbying for blind person's rights throughout the world. Within months of Herie's election, Secretary-General Pedro Zurita of Spain was involved in a near-fatal car crash outside Casablanca. As a result, virtually all the WBU secretariat support responsibilities fell squarely on Herie's office at the CNIB for Marjeram and other staff to handle.

One of his most memorable successes came in 1999. Herie had arrived in Beijing, China, to address a congress of the Universal Postal Union (UPU), and the night before he was scheduled to speak he received a telephone call advising that a proposal had been submitted to the congress that threatened to eliminate free provision of special services for literature for the blind around the world.

Herie and Homer drafted a two-page statement which they dictated line by line to a young Chinese woman. This document, as distributed to the UPU delegates, became a cornerstone of WBU policy. Following Herie's impassioned and effective speech, the proposal was defeated by three votes, ensuring that blind people would continue to receive postal services at no cost to them.

At the beginning of his presidency Herie had chosen "The Power of the Dream," borrowed from the 1996 summer Olympics in Atlanta, Georgia, as the theme for his four-year term. "The power of the dream will be discovered in a future where fairness, equality, and personal freedom will allow the blind of the world to also compete on a level playing field on terms and conditions common to all," he said in his inaugural address.

To mark the end of his term, at the fifth general assembly, held in Melbourne, Australia, in 2000, Herie challenged Terry Kelly, an award-winning blind musician from Nova Scotia, to write and perform a song called "The Power of the Dream," which would capture the spirit and poignancy of his message.

"I can tell you that when Terry performed that song at the closing ceremony of the Melbourne Assembly, it was a showstopper," he said. When released commercially, "The Power of the Dream" was the first CD in the world to feature braille in the liner notes.

At the end of his presidency, in 2000, Herie was voted a lifetime membership in the WBU.

THE CNIB 1996–2001

In 1997, following recommendations in a report prepared for the CNIB by an outside consulting firm, senior management was restructured. Positions were creat-ed for three corporate officers (president, secretary, and treasurer) and three vice-presidents (marketing, communications, and foundations; operations and strategic planning; and client services and technology.)

Barbara Marjeram was appointed corporate secretary in her own right, elevating a woman from the role of administrative assistant to an officer. At the time Herie became managing director, there were few women in senior positions; by the time he left, seven of the ten executive directors were women.

The other major change was reducing the general council from a group of forty-six people to a more manageable eighteen and renaming it the Board of Directors.

"These changes were a huge rupture from the way things had been done for seventy-five years, but," says Homer, "it was something that needed to be done."

Also during this period the CNIB undertook to re-brand itself and its look. Corporate documents were given a striking yellow, black, and white makeover, using an easy-to-read, large-print font. A new magazine, *CNIB Vision*, was launched and mailed in the reader's preferred format to one hundred thousand clients across Canada.

In September 2000, Fran Cutler of Ottawa became chair of the CNIB, only the second woman and the first vision-impaired woman to hold the post. Cutler worked for the CBC as a producer and director of radio programming for Northern Canada, and later she ran the CBC's employment equity office. During her term the transformation of the CNIB library to the digital production system took place along with a major gift campaign to underwrite the cost. The building of a state-of-the-art, fully accessible national headquarters in Toronto also began. Cutler was passionate about the importance of communication to the viability of the organization and was a tireless advocate for the rights of visually impaired people to be able to access information in the format of their choice.

In 1989, Herie established the office of government relations and international liaison in Ottawa and appointed Jim Sanders the first national director to manage this initiative. Cutler worked closely with successive national directors of government relations, including Vangelis Nikias and Cathy Moore, on matters relating to the definition of blindness for tax concessions, accessibility of air and rail transportation, voting independently, and improving Canadian banknotes so blind or visually impaired people could distinguish denominations.

"Euclid understood the importance of CNIB's advocacy role in breaking down barriers with government departments," said Cutler. "Now, when CNIB calls, government officials and politicians respond."

THE VALUE OF A HANDSHAKE

Brantford, Ontario, as most Canadians know, is home to the Gretzky family. And coincidentally, this city of about eighty-six thousand located one hundred kilometres southwest of Toronto is also home to the W. Ross Macdonald School for the Blind. So if you live in Brantford, you probably know something about blindness because the school has been part of the community's identity since 1872.

And that's the way it was for the Gretzkys, until a chance meeting at an airport changed everything.

Walter Gretzky never tires of describing how his family became involved with the CNIB:

> In 1981, Wayne was at Toronto airport waiting for his ride to Brantford when a group of blind and visually impaired teens came up to him. Surprised that the young people knew who he was by the sound of his voice, Wayne was amazed to discover they were big hockey fans and listened to all the games on television. When he got home, he said, "Dad, we've got to do something to help those kids."

And from that chance beginning developed a relationship that would change the lives of thousands of young Canadians who are blind or visually impaired. Today, the Gretzky family's involvement with the CNIB includes hugely successful golf tournaments, a teen computer camp, and a foundation that provides scholarship funds.

In 1981, just weeks after the chance meeting at the airport, the first Wayne Gretzky Celebrity Sports Classic, a tennis tournament, was held. Because the event had been put together on short notice — in only two months — organizers feared high-profile hockey players might not be able to attend, but their concerns were put to rest as limousines began rolling up to a Brantford tennis club and out stepped Gordie Howe, Bobby Orr, and other legends of Canada's game. Over eleven

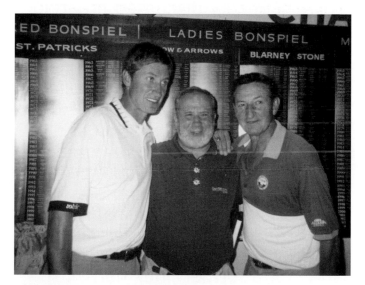

Wayne Gretzky, Euclid Herie, and Walter Gretzky at a CNIB fundraising event.

years, the Celebrity Sports Classic, which turned into a softball tournament that attracted Canadian stars like singer Anne Murray and the late actor John Candy, raised more than $1 million in donations for the CNIB.

In 1990 the CNIB Walter Gretzky Celebrity Golf Tournament, held annually in Brantford, was launched; by 2004 it had become one of the CNIB's premier fundraising events. Other Gretzky golf tournaments are held across Canada.

By the mid-1980s, with the potential of the new technology becoming apparent, Herie and Walter Gretzky discussed creating a learning opportunity for young people. And from a simple handshake between two men of their word began the CNIB Gretzky SCORE (Summer Computer Opportunities in Recreation and Education) Teen Camp, a computer, career, and leadership summer experience for teens who are blind, visually impaired, or deaf-blind. The first SCORE camp was held in Brantford in 1985, and Walter Gretzky, a former linesman with Bell Canada, was so involved with the project that he did the wiring for those early computers himself.

Each summer since then, about twenty blind, visually impaired, and deaf-blind teenagers from across Canada and a few more from around the world arrive in Toronto to work in teams, attend classes, and engage in practical, fun sessions designed to develop skills and increase understanding of the opportunities available to them in the future world of work. Classes are held in a state-of-the-art computer lab located at IBM Canada's headquarters in Markham, Ontario.

The program has gone on to become an international success story boasting graduates from Australia, China, Russia, Japan, Sweden, Germany, New Zealand, Spain, England, Uganda, and the United States. And many of the foreign graduates, especially those from developing countries, have gone on to become leaders in the blindness field in their own right.

More than 350 graduates, all of whom leave with enhanced self-esteem and confidence in their ability to create meaningful lives for themselves, have completed the SCORE program.

A highlight of the camp is always the closing banquet, with

Walter himself as the keynote speaker. Although the SCORE program is available to the participants at no cost to them through sponsorships, the experience is priceless.

In September 1990, the launch of Wayne Gretzky's autobiography marked the first time in the world that a major publication was published simultaneously in print and braille. A portion of the print sales were donated to the CNIB.

In 1993 Walter suffered a near-fatal aneurysm that destroyed a decade of memories and left him with some cognitive difficulties. It could not, however, erase or destroy his boundless compassion or enthusiasm.

The Walter and Wayne Gretzky Scholarship Foundation was established in 1996 to present scholarships to eligible blind and visually impaired students planning to study at the post-secondary level. The value of the scholarships ranges from $3,000 to $5,000, and they are given to as many as twenty deserving students each year. To date, the Gretzkys have raised more than $4 million for their foundation, and when he can, Walter likes to telephone the recipients himself to give them the good news and chat for a few minutes about their goals and dreams.

None of this would have been possible without Ron Finucan, long-time friend of Walter, Wayne, and the Gretzky family, who also happens to be the CNIB's national manager of gift planning and major gifts and corporate development. Finucan carefully manages the relationship with the Gretzkys, ensuring that the family's wishes are carried out while protecting their privacy.

In 1999, Walter and Phyllis Gretzky were presented with the Arthur Napier Magill Distinguished Service Award, the highest award CNIB can give its volunteers. The award not only recognized their role as superb fundraisers but also expressed appreciation for them as distinguished ambassadors for the organization. In 2004, Walter was voted an honorary member of the institute.

The Gretzkys' work with the CNIB has been recognized provincially and nationally. Wayne's Order of Canada citation mentions his work with the CNIB, as does his Order of Ontario.

In 2001, the CNIB district office in Brantford was renamed the CNIB Gretzky Family Service Centre.

WINDING DOWN

In late 2000 Herie announced that he would retire in November 2001. "I hadn't lost my heart or interest for the CNIB but had decided I should retire at sixty-two."

A search for his replacement was begun, and from a field of eighty candidates, the chosen successor was James Sanders, who had been Herie's vice-president of client services and technology. Herie recalled his term of service.

> Looking back, I believe my most bitter disappointment was that I never resolved the issue with the Library of Canada and accessible information for blind people. I wanted the statute of the Library of Canada to be amended to say that it would be the repository and library for the blind in Canada but this never happened. Today, other than the CNIB Library, we do not have a credible library service for blind people in this country. We still don't have a braille press and other than two small independent magazines, all our reading material comes from the U.S. Canada has failed in its public policy to establish equitable library services for the print handicapped and has the dubious distinction of being the only nation in the industrial world not to do so. Sighted Canadians have access to libraries funded from the public purse but blind, or other print disabled Canadians, do not. I never resolved that. My other regret was that I never got braille bills passed in the provincial legislatures mandating a blind student's right to be taught braille.

Some things did go his way, though.

The CNIB had a corporate conscience and we respected our employees. We valued human rights acts. We treated our people with dignity when we closed workshops and residences. In my time we replaced twenty buildings and the communities realized we were still going to be there.

The CNIB was also ahead of its time in adopting sexual harassment in the workplace policies and providing same-sex benefits. We did that before it was required by legislation.

As for my legacy for the CNIB and for blind people in Canada, that's what history has to answer. I'd like to think that we empowered blind people and became more of a community-based organization.

Ultimately, the CNIB followed the Canadian way, and if this book proves nothing else, I hope it shows that CNIB was as much shaped by this country as it played a role in shaping the lives of blind Canadians.

Recognitions over the course of his work include an honorary degree from the University of Manitoba, the Order of Canada in 1998, life membership in the World Blind Union in 2000, and, in 2002, the Ambrose M. Shotwell Award, given by the American-based Association for Education and Rehabilitation of the Blind and Visually Impaired in recognition of an individual whose leadership and services have been influential at an international level.

The award that means the most to him, though, was the Order of the Buffalo Hunt, given to him by his home province of Manitoba in 1995. "When I got the award, the fellow told me the two recipients whose names were directly above mine were Mother Theresa and [former U.S. president] Jimmy Carter, so I was in very good company."

As the tributes began to pour in for a career that exceeded probably even Herie's expectations, dinners and special events were held across the country in his honour.

Gerrard Grace, who held sixteen positions with the CNIB over the course of his long career with CNIB, culminating in vice-president of external relations in 2004, knew Herie well.

"Euclid did many outstanding things during his tenure as CNIB president," Grace said.

> He understood the importance of branding before it was a buzz word. He led the charge to save Louis Braille's birthplace in Coupvray, France, he created a vision for the CNIB that was modern and corporate, he got rid of cronyism and brought high standards of professionalism to the organization, and he took the CNIB to a higher level. He closed buildings that no longer functioned and he got rid of all the shabby offices. His thinking was if we can't afford to be in a decent place, we shouldn't be there at all.
>
> But the greatest thing he did — and I think this is what he will be remembered for — he gave blind people, by example, a sense of purpose, dignity and self-worth that they have never had before. He can take his place with royalty or presidents and his message is very clear: it is respectable to be blind.

In 2001, Herie established the World Braille Foundation to provide braille, braille equipment and technology, teacher training and materials, and other support to groups of blind people and schools for the blind in developing countries. By 2004, twenty-five projects had been funded in China, Africa, South America, India, Cuba, and the Philippines, bringing literacy to thousands.

In lieu of gifts at his retirement, the national and divisional boards made substantial contributions to the foundation; the Alberta-NWT-Nunavut division preferred to establish the Euclid Herie Technical Aids Scholarship and Leadership Awards.

As his retirement date of October 31 neared, a tribute dinner given by the national board was held in Vancouver. The late watercolourist Toni Onley did the invitations, and as a farewell gift, his management team gave him a horse, enabling him to literally ride off into the sunset.

In a farewell interview with noted Canadian journalist Pamela Wallin shortly before she was appointed consul-general to New York, Herie discussed the changes he had seen over his time as CNIB president:

> The CNIB has truly shown the way of the blind to the world. In my time we have gone from an institution that used to put people to bed at night and employed people in workshops. We gave Canadians, including myself, huge opportunities because when I worked for the CNIB in 1956 there was no

alternative for a young blind person.

Today, all that has changed. In communities in every part of this country CNIB has been a big part of that transition. We have helped change the attitudes of sighted people towards blind people and made some progress, but that's going to be part of another generation.

Attitudes are barriers but through having all blind children in regular schools, working age adults employed in hundreds of different jobs, and enabling seniors to continue to do the things they enjoy, we have shown that blind people can live independent, meaningful lives.

Changing what it means to be blind is something I had to change in myself, first. Then we set about to change what it means for blind women who have no value or status

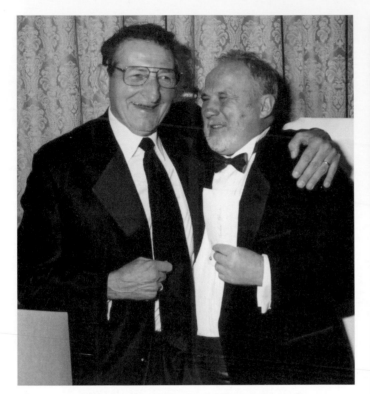

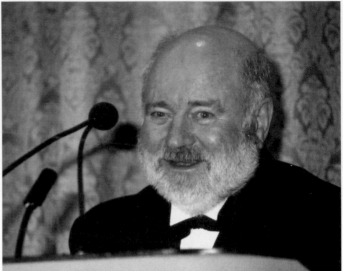

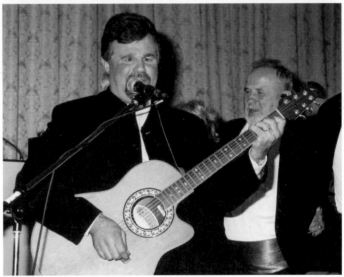

in most countries of the world, and for all the blind children not in school today because there is no brailler or paper for them.

I hope I have shown by example that a blind person can be part of what's going on in the world. When I was younger, I didn't understand that it's respectable to be blind

Walter Gretzky (top left), the late Toni Onley (top right), and Terry Kelly (bottom right) at Euclid Herie's retirement party in Vancouver.

AFTERWORD

At 8:30 a.m. on September 11, 2001, I convened my final session with the CNIB's national management group at the Kempenfelt Conference Centre on Lake Simcoe, Barrie, north of Toronto. Seventy-five people, most of them women, from sixty-five offices across Canada made up the senior executive and operations teams. The previous evening we had shared a retirement tribute and farewell that had included the presentation of a horse and saddle as an imaginative and generous parting gift.

Katherine Calleja, my personal assistant, had driven up from Toronto that morning so I could leave the meeting as soon as I had handed it over to my successor, Jim Sanders, who would become president and CEO of the CNIB on November 1. As Katherine and I drove out of the park, she said, "Dr. Herie, I think a plane just flew into the World Trade Center in New York!"

Minutes later, driving south on Highway 400, we heard of the second, third, and fourth horrific incidents. The range and depth of personal emotions at saying good-bye to close colleagues and friends was tempered by that morning's events and the moments of infamy that would redraw the human map for all time.

More than three years have passed since that day, time enough to reflect on life and events at the CNIB post–Euclid Herie.

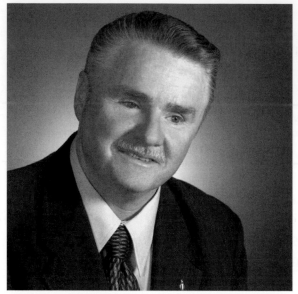

Jim Sanders.

NEW LEADERSHIP, NEW BUILDING

James W. Sanders was born on March 14, 1947, in Thunder Bay, Ontario, the second of eleven children. I once asked, for no particular reason, what the "W" stood for. Jim replied that it stood for Wootten, a name that has been in the Sanders family since 1535. Interestingly, the first Wootten Sanders had been left visually impaired when he was hit by a horse and cart in a London lane.

Severely visually impaired from birth, Jim began his association with the CNIB at two months of age, when he was registered by administrator Norm Gilbey, who became Jim's early mentor. Unlike

most children his age who were blind or visually impaired, Jim did not attend the School for the Blind in Brantford. Long before educational mainstreaming was common, he attended public schools. By age sixteen he worked part-time at the local hospital's Smoke Shoppe, and at twenty he was working summers at the Lake Joseph Centre, where he met and eventually married Anne Wooding, a teacher. Jim graduated from Thunder Bay's Lakehead University in 1969.

Jim began his formal career with the CNIB in CaterPlan, where he worked for two years and then, in a somewhat unusual career move, transferred into the public relations department. "Until then," he said, "CaterPlan had me." In 1979, he moved to the Alberta division, where he became executive director in 1983. His next move took him to British Columbia at the same level in 1985. A few years later, the CNIB decided to establish a permanent, high-profile presence in Ottawa to manage national and international issues and programs, so Jim, who is bilingual, Anne, and their twin daughters moved there in 1989.

In 1997, Jim was appointed vice-president of client services and international relations, and the family moved to Toronto. CNIB national chair Gary Homer had led a seven-member committee to search for the new president and, for the first time, a professional recruiting firm was engaged to direct the search. Some eighty candidates are said to have been considered and in August 2001, the National Board voted to appoint Jim Sanders president and chief executive officer.

Jim's goal for almost thirty years to become first among equals had become a reality.

Besides his role as president of the CNIB, Jim is also executive director of the War Blinded Association and a former officer of the World Blind Union. In 2004 he was named to the Order of Canada.

The board also appoints two other paid officers: corporate secretary and treasurer and chief financial officer. Both positions report to the president, with corporate and fiduciary responsibilities to the board. Barbara Marjeram, who was born in London, England, and came to Canada at age thirty, joined the CNIB staff in 1990 and is the current corporate secretary. Marjeram, like her predecessors (formerly known as recording secretaries), is the organizational link to the president's office and also for the chair and board, ensuring a massive paper and information flow that at times risks crushing the corporate entity. Craig Lillico, a native of Peterborough, Ontario was appointed to his position as treasurer in April 2001, a few months before I retired.

On the morning of November 1, 2001, my first day of retirement, I received a phone call from Jim. After past and present presidents had exchanged greetings, he told me that his first priority would be to sign the documents for the sale of CNIB land, the profits of which would be used to finance the construction of a state-of-the-art building on the BakerWood site at 1929 Bayview Avenue in Toronto. Lillico, already buried in significant financial issues and a dramatic policy change on revenue sharing, would spend the next three years directing the entire building project and interim relocation for the institute's operations in Toronto.

The new building, which opened as scheduled in 2004, features 13,000 square metres of space over a 2,323-square-metre parking facility. With its wide hallways, open concept design, talking elevators, and modern efficiencies, the building will allow the CNIB to deliver enhanced services and to better manage administrative, research, and planning functions. Long gone are the residence, workshops, CaterPlan, and dungeon storage areas. The library, hidden down a long hallway in the old building, is now one of the first things a visitor to the new building sees. The building will allow better production of braille, distribution of technical aids, and delivery of rehabilitation services to a discerning clientele. The new building resonates with the bustle of CNIB staff, blind, visually impaired, and sighted, going about their workdays — just as the old building did. Fully accessible, this building will serve as a model of visionary architectural and engineering designs for Canada and elsewhere.

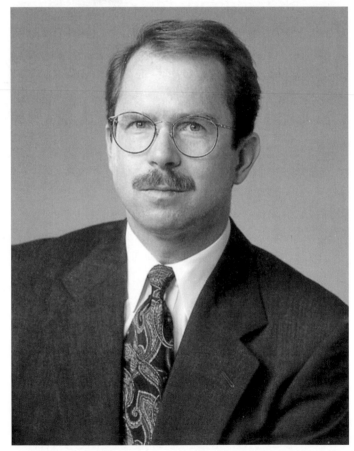

Craig Lillico.

All six of us who preceded Sanders in the top job over eighty-three years shared two things in common: we were all men and we were all clients of the institute. Age, education, background, and residency varied, as did our length of time in office. Four of us retired from the position; Holmes and Mercer left to pursue other successful careers. But what has been remarkable throughout this journey to independence has been the similarity, the almost predictability, of the issues and priorities we have faced, including trying to keep up with the expanding numbers of blind and visually impaired Canadians seeking increasingly complex services.

In 2003, the same year he retired from a lifelong career with the Bank of Nova Scotia, Richard (Dick) Hale-Sanders was elected the CNIB's fourteenth chair. Dick had earlier chaired the Ontario division and served on the national finance committee. Born in Montreal, he had been acquainted with the CNIB since the age of ten because he had an uncle who worked there.

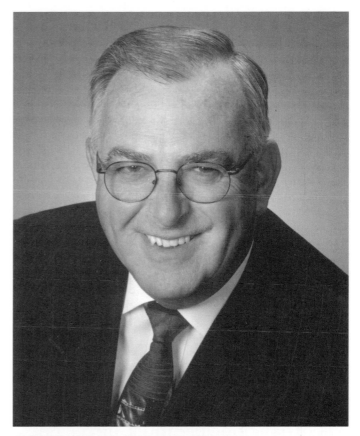

Richard Hale-Sanders.

POLITICAL WILL

In each era, in each generation, what has played out at the CNIB has been a delicate balancing act between trying to deliver high-quality service to clients and working with limited human and financial resources.

On reflection, what strikes me is that the CNIB, with all its turmoil and shortcomings over the years, has never wavered in its objective of providing the quality services demanded by the time and circumstances. Shrewd financial management, including significant debt load at times, has ensured a strong annual operating budget and a healthy balance sheet. Having a client in the president's office results in service standards that remain high.

What sets the CNIB apart from most Canadian charities, however, especially those in the disability field, has been the political will and internal generosity that permits the organization to share resources, in whatever form, to benefit all clients, wherever they choose to live. That principle must never be compromised. Until about twenty years ago, 80 percent of the CNIB's funding came from the government, and the organization raised the rest of the funds. Now, with its annual budget reaching the $100 million level, the 80-20 formula is completely reversed, and the organization must raise 80 percent of its funding. So the CNIB certainly qualifies as a private charity.

In the past decade, civil society and the courts have moved toward good governance and transparency. I believe that the CNIB is well positioned on both accounts. However, the board created in 1997 to replace an unwieldy council of forty-six members has struggled because the CNIB has not found a way to include its clients in matters of governance and policy formation. I, along with others, argued wrongly that the existing structure was the preferable approach. Consolidation and centralization of budgetary and operating functions were long overdue and were achieved with great difficulty. The emerging challenge is to retain grassroots strengths and a viable presence as the shift returns to a Toronto focal point.

The time has also come to repair the basic flaw in funding the library services. That answer is twofold: resolve the internal funding issues and return to a happier time when library services were not a continal source of controversy and division but rather were a flagship service in a fleet of equal flagship services. All must be reminded of Edgar Freel Robinson's vision and generosity a century ago in sharing his private braille collection. However achieved, blind Canadians deserve more equitable access to print. I say more equitable because it will never be truly equal no matter what is achieved. That principle points squarely to the government sector. Empty promises result in empty bookshelves. The beggar's mantra must be replaced with a confident, solid strategy within a defined time frame. We have heard our last empty promise. For far too long, we the blind have stood outside sealed doors to accessible information. We remain hostages to elected officials and a bureaucratic will rooted in inaction and ancient prejudices. If need be, we must invoke — yes, resources do exist to do just that — the rights provided in the Charter and guaranteed by the courts in Canada. The time is yesterday.

BENCH STRENGTH

Featured in this book is a mere sampling of the blind men and women who, as individuals or as part of a professional team, built, shaped, directed, and delivered services within CNIB. The field for recruitment and training was fertile, and in the early years employment offers were often the only game in town. All that has now changed, and it happened slowly and quietly over the past generation. More than ever, the CNIB finds itself competing for the best and brightest among this group of potential staff and volunteers. If the long-standing and successful practice of attracting this calibre of individuals is desirable, and I suggest it is, new, far more creative approaches will be required. Today and tomorrow, it's all about choice, real choice, and that also means choices for the CNIB as an employer, a service agent, and an exciting, progressive environment that assures career growth and enhancement.

On a closing note, I decided not to comment or speculate on the long-term structure of the institute. Fifty years ago we had a managing director and two vice-presidents; one for Western Canada and one for Eastern Canada. Baker held authority for both national and central Canada. Sixty years later, the same model may well prevail. Governance structures and board composition has changed and will continue to change. What appears to have worked well is the close confidence between the president and the chair. From Baker's time this teamwork style provided strong and effective leadership for staff and volunteers. Simply put, my approach was "I promise to run the railroad if you promise to chair the board." In two cases serious issues arose when this special relationship and mutual respect and confidence failed.

Often during my years at the CNIB I tried to explain the corporate culture and internal chemistry that is the very nature of the CNIB's great success and fascinating story in Canadian philanthropy. People asked why we enjoy the reputation and respect of organizations worldwide, why we won the SAP/Stevie Wonder Vision award as a role model organization chosen from some sixty nominees by an international peer review process in 1999. My only and final answer, without equivocation or apology, can best be discovered in this *Journey to Independence*.

Bonne chance et merci.

ADDITIONAL SOURCES

ARCHIVES
National Archives of Canada
The Canadian National Institute for the Blind

NEWSPAPERS
The *Toronto Star*
The *Globe and Mail*

PAPERS, ESSAYS, THESIS
Cowan, Louise. "Home Teaching in Canada: A Rehabilitation Service for Blind Persons." 1948.
Liggett, Margaret, "Unknown Paths." c.1956.
Nichols, Christine M. "The Employment and Occupational Status of the Blind in Canada." 1979.

BOOKS
Catran, Ken and Penny Hansen. *Pioneering a Vision, A History of The Royal New Zealand Foundation for the Blind 1890–1990*. Royal New Zealand Foundation for the Blind, 1992.
Judith M. Dixon (Ed.). *Braille into the Next Millenium*. Washington, DC: The National Libraries for Blind and Physically Handicapped Individuals in North America.

Kitz, Janet F. *Shattered City: The Halifax Explosion and The Road to Recovery*. Nimbus Publishing Ltd., 1989.

MacKay, Donald. *The Square Mile. Merchant Princes of Montreal*. Toronto: Douglas & McIntyre, 1987.

Sewell, Ray and Gloria Sewell, as told to Renate Wilson. *House Without Windows.* Toronto: Peter Martin Associates Limited, 1974.

Trites, Shirley J. *Reading Hands: The Halifax School for the Blind*. Vision Press, 2003.

Wilkins Campbell, Marjorie. *No Compromise.* Toronto: McClelland and Stewart, 1965.

INDEX